I.
TOO MUCH NATURAL HISTORY.

Lord Melbourne, speaking of the fine ladies in London who were fond of talking about their ailments, used to complain that they gave him too much of their natural history. There are a good many writers—usually men—who, with the best intentions, discuss woman as if she had merely a physical organization, and as if she existed only for one object, the production and rearing of children. Against this some protest may well be made.

Doubtless there are few things more important to a community than the health of its women. The Sandwich-Island proverb says:—

> "If strong is the frame of the mother,
> The son will give laws to the people."

And, in nations where all men give laws, all men need mothers of strong frames.

Moreover, there is no harm in admitting that all the rules of organization are imperative; that soul and body, whether of man or woman, are made in harmony, so that each part of our nature must accept the limitations of the other. A man's soul may yearn to the stars; but so long as the body cannot jump so high, he must accept the body's veto. It is the same with any veto interposed in advance by the physical structure of woman. Nobody objects to this general principle. It is only when clerical gentlemen or physiological gentlemen undertake to go a step farther, and put in that veto on their own responsibility, that it is necessary to say, "Hands off, gentlemen! Precisely because women are women, they, not you, are to settle that question."

One or two points are clear. Every specialist is liable to overrate his own specialty; and the man who thinks of woman only as a wife and mother is apt to forget, that, before she was either of these, she was a human being. "Women, as such," says an able writer, "are constituted for purposes of maternity and the continuation of mankind." Undoubtedly, and so were men, as such, constituted for paternity. But very much depends on what relative importance we assign to the phrase, "as such." Even an essay so careful, so moderate, and so free from coarseness, as that here quoted, suggests, after all, a slight one-sidedness,—perhaps a natural re-action from the one-sidedness of those injudicious reformers who allow themselves to speak slightingly of "the merely animal function of child-bearing." Higher than either—wiser than both put together—is that noble statement with which Jean Paul begins his fine essay on the education of girls in "Levana." "Before being a wife or mother, one is a human being; and neither motherly nor wifely destination can overbalance or replace the human, but must become its means, not end. As above the poet, the painter, or the hero, so above the mother, does the human being rise pre-eminent."

Here is sure anchorage. We can hold to this. And, fortunately, all the analogies of nature sustain this position. Throughout nature the laws of sex rule everywhere; but they rule a kingdom of their own, always subordinate to the greater kingdom of the vital functions. Every creature, male or female, finds in its sexual relations only a subordinate part of its existence. The need of food, the need of exercise, the joy of living, these come first, and absorb the bulk of its life, whether the individual be male or female. This *Antiope* butterfly, that flits at this moment past my window,—the first of the season,—spends almost all its existence in a form where the distinction of sex lies dormant: a few days, I might almost say a few hours, comprise its whole sexual consciousness, and the majority of its race die before reaching that epoch. The law of sex is written absolutely through the whole insect world. Yet everywhere it is written as a secondary and subordinate law. The life which is common to the sexes is the principal life; the life which each sex leads, "as such," is a minor and subordinate thing.

The same rule pervades nature. Two riders pass down the street before my window. One rides a horse, the other a mare. The animals were perhaps foaled in the same stable, of the same progenitors. They have been reared alike, fed alike, trained alike, ridden alike; they need the same exercise, the same grooming; nine tenths of their existence are the same, and only the other tenth is different. Their whole organization is marked by the distinction of sex: but, though the marking is ineffaceable, the distinction is not the first or most important fact.

If this be true of the lower animals, it is far more true of the higher. The mental and moral laws of the universe touch us first and chiefly as human beings. We eat our breakfasts as human beings, not as men and women; and it is the same with nine tenths of our interests and duties in life. In legislating or philosophizing for woman, we must neither forget that she has an organization distinct from that of man, nor must we exaggerate the fact. Not "first the womanly and then the human," but first the human and then the womanly, is to be the order of her training.

II.
DARWIN, HUXLEY, AND BUCKLE.

When any woman, old or young, asks the question, Which among all modern books ought I to read first? the answer is plain. She should read Buckle's lecture before the Royal Institution upon "The Influence of Woman on the Progress of Knowledge." It is one of two papers contained in a thin volume called "Essays by Henry Thomas Buckle." As a means whereby a woman may become convinced that her sex has a place in the intellectual universe, this little essay is almost indispensable. Nothing else takes its place.

Darwin and Huxley seem to make woman simply a lesser man, weaker in body and mind,—an affectionate and docile animal, of inferior grade. That there is any aim in the distinction of the sexes, beyond the perpetuation of the race, is nowhere recognized by them, so far as I know. That there is any thing in the intellectual sphere to correspond to the physical difference; that here also the sexes are equal yet diverse, and the natural completion and complement of the other,—this neither Huxley nor Darwin explicitly recognizes. And with the utmost admiration for their great teachings in other ways, I must think that here they are open to the suspicion of narrowness.

Huxley wrote in "The Reader," in 1864, a short paper called "Emancipation—Black and White," in which, while taking generous ground in behalf of the legal and political position of woman, he yet does it pityingly, *de haut en bas*, as for a creature hopelessly inferior, and so heavily weighted already by her sex, that she should be spared all further trials. Speaking through an imaginary critic, who seems to represent himself, he denies "even the natural equality of the sexes," and declares "that in every excellent character, whether mental or physical, the average woman is inferior to the average man, in the sense of having that character less in quantity and lower in quality." Finally he goes so far as "to defend the startling paradox that even in physical beauty, man is the superior." He admits that for a brief period of early youth the case may be doubtful, but claims that after thirty the superior beauty of man is unquestionable. Thus reasons Huxley; the whole essay being included in his volume of "Lay Sermons, Addresses, and Reviews."[1]

[1]. Pp. 22, 23, Am. ed.

Darwin's best statements on the subject may be found in his "Descent of Man."[2] He is, as usual, more moderate and guarded than Huxley. He says, for instance: "It is generally admitted that with women the powers of intuition, of rapid perception, and perhaps of imitation, are more strongly marked than in man; but some, at least, of these faculties are characteristic of the lower races, and therefore of a past and lower state of civilization." Then he passes to the usual assertion that man has thus far attained to a higher eminence than woman. "If two lists were made of the most eminent men and women in poetry, painting, sculpture, music,—comprising composition and performance,—history, science, and philosophy, with half a dozen names under each subject, the two lists would not bear comparison." But the obvious answer, that nearly every name on his list, upon the masculine side, would probably be taken from periods when woman was excluded from any fair competition,—this he does not seem to recognize at all. Darwin, of all men, must admit that superior merit generally arrives later, not earlier, on the scene; and the question for him to answer is, not whether woman equalled man in the first stages of the intellectual "struggle for life," but whether she is not gaining on him now.@

[2]. II., 311, Am. Ed.

If, in spite of man's enormous advantage in the start, woman has already overtaken his very best performances in several of the highest intellectual departments,—as, for instance, prose fiction and dramatic representation,—then it is mere dogmatism in Mr. Darwin to deny that she may yet do the same in other departments. We in this generation have actually seen this success achieved by Rachel and Ristori in the one art, by "George Sand" and "George Eliot" in the other. Woman is, then, visibly gaining on man, in the sphere of intellect; and, if so, Mr. Darwin, at least, must accept the inevitable inference.

But this is arguing the question on the superficial facts merely. Buckle goes deeper, and looks to principles. That superior quickness of women, which Darwin dismisses so lightly as something belonging to savage epochs, is to Buckle the sign of a quality which he holds essential, not only to literature and art, but to science itself. Go among ignorant women, he says, and you will find them more quick and intelligent than equally ignorant men. A woman will usually tell you the way in the street more readily than a man can; a woman can always understand a foreigner more easily; and Dr. Currie says in his letters, that when a laborer and his wife came to consult him, he always got all the information from the wife. Buckle illustrates this at some length, and points out that a woman's mind is by its nature deductive and quick; a man's mind, inductive and slow; that each has its value, and that science profoundly needs both.

"I will endeavor," he says, "to establish two propositions. First, that women naturally prefer the deductive method to the inductive. Secondly, that women, by encouraging in men deductive habits of thought, have rendered an immense though unconscious service to the progress of science, by preventing scientific investigators from being as exclusively inductive as they would otherwise be."

Then he shows that the most important scientific discoveries of modern times—as of the law of gravitation by Newton, the law of the forms of crystals by Haüy, and the metamorphosis of plants by Goethe—were all essentially the results of that *a priori* or deductive method, "which, during the last two centuries, Englishmen have unwisely despised." They were all the work, in a manner, of the imagination,—of the intuitive or womanly quality of mind. And nothing can be finer or truer than the words in which Buckle predicts the benefits that are to come from the intellectual union of the sexes for the work of the future. "In that field which we and our posterity have yet to traverse, I firmly believe that the imagination will effect quite as much as the understanding. Our poetry will have to re-enforce our logic, and we must feel quite as much as we must argue. Let us, then, hope that the imaginative and emotional minds of one sex will continue to accelerate the great progress by acting upon and improving the colder and harder minds of the other sex. By this coalition, by this union of different faculties, different tastes, and different methods, we shall go on our way with the greater ease."

III.
WHICH IS THE STRONGER?

What is strength,—the brute hardness of iron, or the more delicate strength of steel? Which is the stronger,—the physical frame that can strike the harder blow, or that which can endure the greater strain and yet last longer? "Man can lift a heavier weight," says a writer on physiology, "but woman can watch more enduringly at the bedside of her sick child." The strain upon the system of all women who have borne and reared children is as great in its way as that upon the system of the carpenter or the woodchopper; and the power to endure it is as properly to be called strength.

Again, which is the stronger in the domain of will,—the man who carries his points by energy and command, or the woman who carries hers by patience and persuasion? the man in the household who leads and decides, or the woman who foresees, guards, manages? the mother of the family, who puts the commas and semicolons in her children's lives, as Jean Paul Richter says, or the father who puts in the colons and periods? It may be hard to say which type of strength is the more to be admired, but it is clear that they are both genuine types.

One grows tired of hearing young men who can do nothing but row, or swing dumb-bells, and are thrown wholly "off their training" by the loss of a night's sleep, speak contemptuously of the physical weakness of a woman who can watch with a sick person half a dozen nights together. It is absurd to hear a man who is prostrated by a single reverse in business speak of being "encumbered" with a wife who can perhaps alter the habits of a lifetime more easily than he can abandon his half-dollar cigars. It is amusing to read the criticisms of languid and graceful masculine essayists on the want of vigorous intellect in the sex that wrote "Aurora Leigh" and "Middlemarch" and "Consuelo."

It may be that a man's strength is not a woman's, or a woman's strength that of a man. I am arguing for equivalence, not identity. The greater part played in the phenomena of woman's strength by sensibility and impulse and variations and tears—this does not affect the matter. What I have never been able to see is, that woman as such is, in the long-run and tried by all the tests, a weaker being than man. And it would seem that any man, in proportion as he lives longer and sees more of life, must have the conceit taken out of him by actual contact with some woman—be she mother, sister, wife, daughter, or friend—who is not only as strong as himself in all substantial regards, but it may be, on the whole, a little stronger.

IV.
THE SPIRIT OF SMALL TYRANNY.

When Mr. John Smauker and the Bath footmen invited Sam Weller to their "swarry," consisting of a boiled leg of mutton, each guest had some expression of contempt and wrath for the humble little greengrocer who served them,—"in the true spirit," Dickens says, "of the very smallest tyranny." The very fact that they were subject to being ordered about in their own persons gave them a peculiar delight in issuing tyrannical orders to others: just as sophomores in college torment freshmen because other sophomores once teased the present tormentors themselves; and Irishmen denounce the Chinese for underbidding them in the labor-market, precisely as they were themselves denounced by native-born Americans thirty years ago. So it has sometimes seemed to me that the men whose own positions and claims are really least commanding are those who hold most resolutely that women should be kept in their proper place of subordination.

A friend of mine maintains the theory that men large and strong in person are constitutionally inclined to do justice to women, as fearing no competition from them in the way of bodily strength; but that small and weak men are apt to be vehemently opposed to any thing like equality in the sexes. He quotes in defence of his theory the big soldier in London who justified himself for allowing his little wife to chastise him, on the ground that it pleased her and did not hurt him; and on the other hand cites the extreme domestic tyranny of the dwarf Quilp. He declares that in any difficult excursion among woods and mountains, the guides and the able-bodied men are often willing to have women join the party, while it is sure to be opposed by those who doubt their own strength or are reluctant to display their weakness. It is not necessary to go so far as my friend goes; but many will remember some fact of this kind, making such theories appear not quite so absurd as at first.

Thus it seems from the "Life and Letters" of Sydney Dobell, the English poet, that he was opposed both to woman suffrage and woman authorship, believing the movement for the former to be a "blundering on to the perdition of womanhood." It appears that against all authorship by women his convictions yearly grew stronger, he regarding it as "an error and an anomaly." It seems quite in accordance with my friend's theory to hear, after this, that Sydney Dobell was slight in person and a life-long invalid; nor is it surprising, on the same theory, that his poetry took no deep root, and that it will not be likely to survive long, except perhaps in his weird ballad of "Ravelston." But he represents a large class of masculine intellects, of secondary and mediocre quality, whose opinions on this subject are not so much opinions as instinctive prejudices against a competitor who may turn out their superior. Whether they know it, or not, their aversion to the authorship of women is very much like the conviction of a weak pedestrian, that women are not naturally fitted to take long walks; or the opinion of a man whose own accounts are in a muddle, that his wife is constitutionally unfitted to understand business.

It is a pity to praise either sex at the expense of the other. The social inequality of the sexes was not produced so much by the voluntary tyranny of man, as by his great practical advantage at the outset; human history necessarily beginning with a period when physical strength was sole ruler. It is unnecessary, too, to consider in how many cases women may have justified this distrust; and may have made themselves as obnoxious as Horace Walpole's maids of honor, whose coachman left his savings to his son on condition that he should never marry a maid of honor. But it is safe to say that on the whole the feeling of contempt for women, and the love to exercise arbitrary power over them, is the survival of a crude impulse which the world is outgrowing, and which is in general least obvious in the manliest men. That clear and able English writer, Walter Bagehot, well describes "the contempt for physical weakness and for women which marks early society. The non-combatant population is sure to fare ill during the ages of combat. But these defects, too, are cured or lessened; women have now marvellous means of winning their way in the world; and mind without muscle has far greater force than muscle without mind."[3]

[3]. Physics and Politics, p. 79.

V.
"THENOBLESEX."

A highly educated American woman of my acquaintance once employed a French tutor in Paris, to assist her in teaching Latin to her little grandson. The Frenchman brought with him a Latin grammar, written in his own language, with which my friend was quite pleased, until she came to a passage relating to the masculine gender in nouns, and claiming grammatical precedence for it on the ground that the male sex is the noble sex,—"*le sexe noble*." "Upon that," she said, "I burst forth in indignation, and the poor teacher soon retired. But I do not believe," she added, "that the Frenchman has the slightest conception, up to this moment, of what I could find in that phrase to displease me."

I do not suppose he could. From the time when the Salic Law set French women aside from the royal succession, on the ground that the kingdom of France was "too noble to be ruled by a woman," the claim of nobility has been all on one side. The State has strengthened the Church in this theory, the Church has strengthened the State; and the result of all is, that French grammarians follow both these high authorities. When even the good Père Hyacinthe teaches, through the New York Independent, that the husband is to direct the conscience of his wife, precisely as the father directs that of his child, what higher philosophy can you expect of any Frenchman than to maintain the claims of "*lesexenoble* "?

We see the consequence, even among the most heterodox Frenchmen. Rejecting all other precedents and authorities, the poor Communists still held to this. Consider, for instance, this translation of a marriage-contract under the Commune, which lately came to light in a trial reported in the "Gazette des Tribunaux:"—

FRENCHREPUBLIC.

The citizen Anet, son of Jean Louis Anet, and the *citoyenne* Maria Saint; she engaged to follow the said citizen everywhere and to love him always.—ANET. MARIA SAINT.

Witnessed by the under-mentioned citizen and *citoyenne*.—FOURIER. LAROCHE.

PARIS, April 22, 1871.

What a comfortable arrangement is this! Poor *citoyenne* Maria Saint, even when all human laws have suspended their action, still holds by her grammar, still must annex herself to *le sexe noble*. She still must follow citizen Anet as the feminine pronoun follows the masculine, or as a verb agrees with its nominative case in number and in person. But with what a lordly freedom from all obligation does citizen Anet, representative of this nobility of sex, accept the allegiance! The citizeness may "follow him," certainly,—so long as she is not in the way,—and she must "love him always;" but he is not bound. Why should he be? It would be quite ungrammatical.

Yet, after all is said and done, there is a brutal honesty in this frank subordination of the woman according to the grammar. It has the same merit with the old Russian marriage-consecration: "Here, wolf, take thy lamb," which at least put the thing clearly, and made no nonsense about it. I do not know that anywhere in France the wedding ritual is now so severely simple as that, but I know that in some rural villages of that country the bride is still married in a mourning-gown. I should think she would be.

VI.
PHYSIOLOGICAL CROAKING.

A very old man once came to King Agis of Sparta, to lament over the degeneracy of the times. The king replied, "What you say must be true; for I remember that when I was a boy, I heard my father say that when he was a boy, he heard my grandfather say the same thing."

It is a sufficient answer to most of the croakers, that doubtless the same things have been said in every generation since the beginning of recorded time. Till within twenty years, for instance, it has been the accepted theory, that civilized society lost in vigor what it gained in refinement. This is now generally admitted to be a delusion growing out of the fact that civilization keeps alive many who would have died under barbarism. These feebler persons enter into the average, and keep down the apparent health of the community; but it is the triumph of civilization that they exist at all. I am inclined to think, that when we come to compare the nineteenth century with the seventeenth, as regards the health of women and the size of families, we shall find much the same result.

We look around us, and see many invalid or childless women. We say the Pilgrim mothers were not like these. We cheat ourselves by this perpetual worship of the pioneer grandmother. How the young bachelors, who write dashing articles in the newspapers, denounce their "nervous" sisters, for instance, and belabor them with cruel memories of their ancestors! "The great-grandmother of this helpless creature, very likely, was a pioneer in the woods; reared a family of twelve or thirteen children; spun, scrubbed, wove, and cooked; lived to eighty-five, with iron muscles, a broad chest and keen, clear eyes." But no one can study the genealogies of our older New England families without noticing how many of the aunts and sisters and daughters of this imaginary Amazon died young. I think there may be the same difference between the households of to-day and the Puritan households that there is confessedly between the American families and the Irish: fewer children are born, but more survive.

And is it so sure that the families are diminishing, even as respects the number of children born? This is a simple question of arithmetic, for which the materials are being rapidly accumulated by the students of family history. Let each person take the lines of descent which are nearest to himself, to begin with, and compare the number of children born in successive generations. I have, for instance, two such tables at hand, representing two of the oldest New England families, which meet in the same family of children in this generation.

FIRST TABLE.

	CHILDREN
First generation (emigrated 1629)	9
Second generation	7
Third generation	7
Fourth generation	8
Fifth generation	7
Sixth generation	10
Average	8

SECOND TABLE.

	CHILDREN
First generation (emigrated 1636)	10
Second generation	7
Third generation	14
Fourth generation	7
Fifth generation	6
Sixth generation	4
Seventh generation	10
Average	8.29

It will be seen that the last generation exhibits the largest family in the first line, and almost the largest—much beyond the average—in the other.

Now, when we consider the great change in all the habits of living, since the Puritan days, and all the vicissitudes to which a single line is exposed,— a whole household being sometimes destroyed by a single hereditary disease,—this is certainly a fair exhibit. These two genealogies were taken at random, because they happened to be nearest at hand. But I suspect any extended examination of genealogies, either of the Puritan families of New England, or the Dutch families of New York, would show much the same result. Some of the descendants of the old Stuyvesant race, for instance, exhibit in this generation a physical vigor which it is impossible that the doughty governor himself could have surpassed.

There are undoubtedly many moral and physiological sins committed, tending to shorten and weaken life; but the progress of knowledge more than counterbalances them. No man of middle age can look at a class of students from our older colleges without seeing them to be physically superior to the same number of college boys taken twenty-five years ago. The organization of girls being far more delicate and complicated, the same reform reaches them more promptly, but it reaches them at last. The little girls of the present day eat better food, wear more healthful clothing, and breathe more fresh air, than their mothers did. The introduction of india-rubber boots and waterproof cloaks alone has given a fresh lease of life to multitudes of women, who otherwise would have been kept housed whenever there was so much as a sprinkling of rain.

It is desirable, certainly, to venerate our grandmothers; but I am inclined to think, on the whole, that their great-granddaughters will be the best.

VII.
THE TRUTH ABOUT OUR GRANDMOTHERS.

Every young woman of the present generation, so soon as she ventures to have a headache or a set of nerves, is immediately confronted by indignant critics with her grandmother. If the grandmother is living, the fact of her existence is appealed to: if there is only a departed grandmother to remember, the maiden is confronted with a ghost. That ghost is endowed with as many excellences as those with which Miss Betsey Trotwood endowed the niece that never had been born; and, as David Copperfield was reproached with the virtues of his unborn sister who "would never have run away," so that granddaughter with the headache is reproached with the ghostly perfections of her grandmother, who never had a headache—or, if she had, it is luckily forgotten. It is necessary to ask, sometimes, what was really the truth about our grandmothers? Were they such models of bodily perfection as is usually claimed?

If we look at the early colonial days, we are at once met by the fact, that although families were then often larger than is now common, yet this phenomenon was by no means universal, and was balanced by a good many childless homes. Of this any one can satisfy himself by looking over any family history; and he can also satisfy himself of the fact,—first pointed out, I believe, by Mrs. Dall,—that third and fourth marriages were then obviously and unquestionably more common than now. The inference would seem to be, that there is a little illusion about the health of those days, as there is about the health of savage races. In both cases, it is not so much that the average health is greater under less highly civilized conditions, but that these conditions kill off the weak, and leave only the strong. Modern civilized society, on the other hand, preserves the health of many men and women—and permits them to marry, and become parents— who under, the severities of savage life or of pioneer life would have died, and given way to others.

On this I will not dwell; because these good ladies were not strictly our grandmothers, being farther removed. But of those who were our grandmothers,—the women of the Revolutionary and post-Revolutionary epochs,—we happen to have very definite physiological observations recorded; not very flattering, it is true, but frank and searching. What these good women are in the imagination of their descendants, we know. Mrs. Stowe describes them as "the race of strong, hardy, cheerful girls that used to grow up in country places, and made the bright, neat New England kitchens of olden times;" and adds, "This race of women, pride of olden time, is daily lessening; and in their stead come the fragile, easily-fatigued, languid girls of a modern age, drilled in book-learning, ignorant of common things."

What, now, was the testimony of those who saw our grandmothers in the flesh? As it happens, there were a good many foreigners, generally Frenchmen, who came to visit the new Republic during the presidency of Washington. Let us take, for instance, the testimony of the two following.

The Abbé Robin was a chaplain in Rochambeau's army during the Revolution, and wrote thus in regard to the American ladies in his "Nouveau Voyage dans l'Amérique Septentrionale," published in 1782:—

"They are tall and well-proportioned; their features are generally regular; their complexions are generally fair and without color.... At twenty years of age the women have no longer the freshness of youth. At thirty-five or forty they are wrinkled and decrepit. The men are almost as premature."

Again: The Chevalier Louis Félix de Beaujour lived in the United States from 1804 to 1814, as consul-general and *chargé d'affaires*; and wrote a book, immediately after, which was translated into English under the title, "A Sketch of the United States at the Commencement of the Present Century." In this he thus describes American women:—

"The women have more of that delicate beauty which belongs to their sex, and in general have finer features and more expression in their physiognomy. Their stature is usually tall, and nearly all are possessed of a light and airy shape,—the breast high, a fine head, and their color of a dazzling whiteness. Let us imagine, under this brilliant form, the most modest demeanor, a chaste and virginal air, accompanied by those single and unaffected graces which flow from artless nature, and we may have an idea of their beauty; but this beauty fades and passes in a moment. At the age of twenty-five their form changes, and at thirty the whole of their charms have disappeared."

These statements bring out a class of facts, which, as it seems to me, are singularly ignored by some of our physiologists. They indicate that the modification of the American type began early, and was, as a rule, due to causes antedating the fashions or studies of the present day. Here are our grandmothers and great-grandmothers as they were actually seen by the eyes of impartial or even flattering critics. These critics were not Englishmen, accustomed to a robust and ruddy type of women, but Frenchmen, used to a type more like the American. They were not mere hasty travellers; for the one lived here ten years, and the other was stationed for some time at Newport, R.I., in a healthy locality, noted in those days for the beauty of its women. Yet we find it their verdict upon these grandmothers of nearly a hundred years ago, that they showed the same delicate beauty, the same slenderness, the same pallor, the same fragility, the same early decline, with which their granddaughters are now reproached.

In some respects, probably, the physical habits of the grandmothers were better: but an examination of their portraits will satisfy any one that they laced more tightly than their descendants, and wore their dresses lower in the neck; and as for their diet, we have the testimony of another French traveller, Volney, who was in America from 1795 to 1798, that "if a premium were offered for a regimen most destructive to the teeth, the stomach, and the health in general, none could be devised more efficacious for these ends than that in use among this people." And he goes on to give particulars, showing a far worse condition in respect to cookery and diet than now prevails in any decent American society.

We have therefore strong evidence that the essential change in the American type was effected in the last century, not in this. Dr. E. H. Clarke says, "A century does not afford a period long enough for the production of great changes. That length of time could not transform the sturdy German *fräulein* and robust English damsel into the fragile American miss." And yet it is pretty clear that the first century and a half of our colonial life had done just this for our grandmothers. And, if so, our physiologists ought to conform their theories to the facts.

VIII.
THE PHYSIQUE OF AMERICAN WOMEN.

I was talking the other day with a New York physician, long retired from practice, who after an absence of a dozen years in Europe has returned within a year to this country. He volunteered the remark, that nothing had so impressed him since his return as the improved health of Americans. He said that his wife had been equally struck with it; and that they had noticed it especially among the inhabitants of cities, among the more cultivated classes, and in particular among women.

It so happened, that within twenty-four hours almost precisely the same remark was made to me by another gentleman of unusually cosmopolitan experience, and past middle age. He further fortified himself by a similar assertion made him by Charles Dickens, in comparing his second visit to this country with his first. In answer to an inquiry as to what points of difference had most impressed him, Dickens said, "Your people, especially the women, look better fed than formerly."

It is possible that in all these cases the witnesses may have been led to exaggerate the original evil, while absent from the country, and so may have felt some undue re-action on their arrival. One of my informants went so far as to say that he was confident that among his circle of friends in Boston and in London a dinnerparty of half a dozen Americans would outweigh an English party of the same number. Granting this to be too bold a statement, and granting the unscientific nature of all these assertions, they still indicate a probability of their own truth until refuted by facts or balanced by similar impressions on the other side. They are further corroborated by the surprise expressed by Huxley and some other recent Englishmen at finding us a race more substantial than they had supposed.

The truth seems to be, that Nature is endeavoring to take a new departure in the American, and to produce a race more finely organized, more sensitive, more pliable, and of more nervous energy, than the races of Northern Europe; that this change of type involves some risk to health in the process, but promises greater results whenever the new type shall be established. I am confident that there has been within the last twenty years a great improvement in the physical habits of the more cultivated classes, at least, in this country,—better food, better air, better habits as to bathing and exercise. The great increase of athletic games; the greatly increased proportion of seaside and mountain life in summer; the thicker shoes and boots of women and little girls, permitting them to go out more freely in all weathers—these are among the permanent gains. The increased habit of dining late, and of taking only a lunch at noon, is of itself an enormous gain to the professional and mercantile classes, because it secures time for eating and for digestion. Even the furnaces in houses, which seemed at first so destructive to the very breath of life, turn out to have given a new lease to it; and open fires are being rapidly re-introduced as a provision for enjoyment and health, when the main body of the house has been tempered by the furnace. There has been, furthermore, a decided improvement in the bread of the community, and a very general introduction of other farinaceous food. All this has happened within my own memory, and gives *apriori* probability to the alleged improvement in physical condition within twenty years.

And, if these reasonings are still insufficient on the one side, it must be remembered that the facts of the census are almost equally inadequate when quoted on the other. If, for instance, all the young people of a New Hampshire village take a fancy to remove to Wisconsin, it does not show that the race is dying out because their children swell the birth-rate of Wisconsin instead of New Hampshire. If in a given city the births among the foreign-born population are twice as many in proportion as among the American, we have not the whole story until we learn whether the deaths are not twice as many also. If so, the inference is, that the same recklessness brought the children into the world, and sent them out of it; and no physiological inference whatever can be drawn. It was clearly established by the medical commission of the Boston Board of Health, a few years ago, that "the general mortality of the foreign element is much greater than that of the native element of our population." "This is found to be the case," they add, "throughout the United States as well as in Boston."

So far as I can judge, all our physiological tendencies are favorable rather than otherwise: and the transplantation of the English race seems now likely to end in no deterioration, but in a type more finely organized, and more comprehensive and cosmopolitan; and this without loss of health, of longevity, or of physical size and weight. And, if this is to hold true, it must be true not only of men, but of women.

IX.
"VERY MUCH FATIGUED."

The newspapers say that the Wyoming ladies, after their first trial of jury-duty, looked very much fatigued. Well, why not?

Is it not the privilege of their sex to be fatigued? Is it not commonly said to be one of their most becoming traits? "The strength of womanhood lies in its weakness," and so on; and, if emancipation does not destroy this lovely debility, it is not so bad, after all. If a graceful languor is desirable, then the more of it the better. Instead of the women's coming out of the jury-box like Amazons, they simply came out so many tired women. They were not spoiled into strength, but "very much fatigued."

In London or New York, now, this fatigue might have come from six hours of piano-practice, from a day's shopping, from a night's "German." Then the fatigue would be held to be charming and womanly. But to aid in deciding on the guilt or innocence of a fellow-creature, perhaps a fellow-woman,—is that the only pursuit in which fatigue becomes disreputable?

Consider at any rate that in Wyoming Territory these more genteel and feminine forms of fatigue are as yet rare. Pianos are doubtless scarce; in the shops whiskey is the only thing not scarce; "Germans" are uncommon, except in the shape of wandering miners who are looking for other shafts than those of Cupid. Thus cut off from city frivolities, may not the Wyoming ladies be allowed for a while to tire themselves with something useful? Let them have their court duties until good society and "feminine" amusements arrive. Let them at least be serviceable till they can be ornamental—as the English member of Parliament declared that until a man knew which way his interest went, he was justified in temporarily voting according to his conscience.

"Very much fatigued?" How does jury-duty affect men? Is there any thing against which they so fight and struggle? It is recognized by the universal masculine heart as the greatest bore known under civilization. There is nothing which a man will not do in preference. He will go to church twice on a Sunday, he will abjure tobacco for a week, he will over-state his property to the assessor, he will speak respectfully of Congress, he will go without a daily newspaper, he will do any self-devoted and unmasculine thing—if you will only contrive in some way to leave him off the jury-list. If these things are done in the dry tree, what shall be done in the green? That which experienced men hate with this consummation of all hatred, shall inexperienced women endure without fatigue? It is wrong to claim for them such unspeakable superiority.

Look at a jury of men when they re-appear in court after a long detention on a difficult case. What a set of woe-begone wretches they are! What weary eyes, what unkempt hair, what drooping and dilapidated paper collars! Not all the tin wash-basins and soap, not all the crackers and cheese, provided by the gentlemanly sheriff, enable them to look any thing but "very much fatigued." Shall women look more forlorn than these men? No: so long as women are women, they will contrive during the most arduous jury duties to "do up" their hair, they will come provided with unseen relays of fresh cuffs and collars, and out of the most unpromising court-room arrangements they will concoct their cup of tea. Who has not noticed how much better a railway detention or a prolonged trip on a steamboat is borne, in appearance at least, by the women than the men? Fatigued! How did the jury-men look? Probably the jury-women, when they bade his Honor the Judge good-morning, looked incomparably fresher than their companions.

At any rate, when we think what things women endured that they might nurse our sick soldiers, how they had to spend day and night where they might possibly inhale tobacco, probably would hear swearing, and certainly must brave dirt; when we think that they did these things, and were only "very much fatigued,"—why should we fear to risk them in a court-room? Where there is wrong to be righted, innocence to be vindicated, and guilt to be wisely dealt with,—there make room for woman, and she will not shrink from the fatigue. "For thee, fair justice! welcome all," as Sir William Blackstone remarked, when he stopped being a poet and began to be a lawyer.

X.
THE LIMITATIONS OF SEX

Are there any inevitable limitations of sex?

Some reformers, apparently, think that there are not, and that the best way to help woman is to deny the fact of limitations. But I think the great majority of reformers would take a different ground, and would say that the two sexes are mutually limited by nature. They would doubtless add that this very fact is an argument for the enfranchisement of woman: for, if woman is a mere duplicate of man, man can represent her; but if she has traits of her own, absolutely distinct from his, then he cannot represent her, and she must have a voice and a vote of her own.

To this last body of believers I belong. I think that all legal or conventional obstacles should be removed, which debar woman from determining for herself, as freely as man determines, what the real limitations of sex are, and what the merely conventional restriction. But, when all is said and done, there is no doubt that plenty of limitations will remain on both sides.

That man has his limitations, is clear. No matter how finely organized a man may be, how sympathetic, how tender, how loving, there is yet a barrier, never to be passed, that separates the most precious part of the woman's kingdom from him. All the wondrous world of motherhood, with its unspeakable delights, its holy of holies, remains forever unknown by him; he may gaze, but never enter. That halo of pure devotion, which makes a Madonna out of so many a poor and ignorant woman, can never touch his brow. Many a man loves children more than many a woman: but, after all, it is not he who has borne them; to that peculiar sacredness of experience he can never arrive. But never mind whether the loss be a great one or a small one: it is distinctly a limitation; and to every loving mother it is a limitation so important that she would be unable to weigh all the privileges and powers of manhood against this peculiar possession of her child.

Now, if this be true, and if man be thus distinctly limited by the mere fact of sex, can the woman complain that she also should have some natural limitations? Grant that she should have no unnecessary restrictions; and that the course of human progress is constantly setting aside, as needless, point after point that was once held essential. Still, if she finds—as she undoubtedly will find—that natural barriers and hindrances remain at last, and that she can no more do man's whole work in the world than he can do hers, why should she complain? If he can accept his limitations, she must be prepared also to accept hers.

Some of our physiological reformers declare that a girl will be perfectly healthy if she can only be sensibly dressed, and can "have just as much out-door exercise as the boys, and of the same sort, if she choose it." But I have observed that matter a good deal, and have watched the effect of boyish exercise on a good many girls; and I am satisfied that so far from being safely turned loose, as boys can be, they need, for physical health, the constant supervision of wise mothers. Otherwise the very exposure that only hardens the boy may make the girl an invalid for life. The danger comes from a greater sensitiveness of structure,—not weakness, properly so called, since it gives, in certain ways, more power of endurance,—a greater sensitiveness which runs through all a woman's career, and is the expensive price she pays for the divine destiny of motherhood. It is another natural limitation.

No wise person believes in any "reform against Nature," or that we can get beyond the laws of Nature. If I believed the limitations of sex to be inconsistent with woman suffrage for instance, I should oppose this; but I do not see why a woman cannot form political opinions by her baby's cradle, as well as her husband in his workshop, while her very love for the child commits her to an interest in good government. Our duty is to remove all the artificial restrictions we can. That done, it will not be hard for man or woman to acquiesce in the natural limitations.

TEMPERAMENT.

Ἀνδρὸς καὶ γυναικὸς ἡ αὐτὴ ἀρετή.—ANTISTHENES *in Diogenes Laertius,* vi. 1, 5.

"Virtue in man and woman is the same."

XI.
THE INVISIBLE LADY.

The Invisible Lady, as advertised in all our cities a good many years ago, was a mysterious individual who remained unseen, and had apparently no human organs except a brain and a tongue. You asked questions of her, and she made intelligent answers; but where she was, you could no more discover than you could find the man inside the Automaton Chess-Player. Was she intended as a satire on womankind, or as a sincere representation of what womankind should be? To many men, doubtless, she would have seemed the ideal of her sex, could only her brain and tongue have disappeared like the rest of her faculties. Such men would have liked her almost as well as that other mysterious personage on the London sign-board, labelled "The Good Woman," and represented by a female figure without a head.

It is not that any considerable portion of mankind actually wishes to abolish woman from the universe. But the opinion dies hard that she is best off when least visible. These appeals which still meet us for "the sacred privacy of woman" are only the Invisible Lady on a larger scale. In ancient Bœotia, brides were carried home in vehicles whose wheels were burned at the door in token that they would never again be needed. In ancient Rome, it was a queen's epitaph, "She staid at home, and spun,"—*Domum servavit, lanum fecit*. In Turkey, not even the officers of justice can enter the apartments of a woman without her lord's consent. In Spain and Spanish America, the veil replaces the four walls of the house, and is a portable seclusion. To be visible is at best a sign of peasant blood and occupations; to be high-bred is to be invisible.

In the Azores I found that each peasant family endeavored to secure for one or more of its daughters the pride and glory of living unseen. The other sisters, secure in innocence, tended cattle on lonely mountain-sides, or toiled bare-legged up the steep ascents, their heads crowned with orange-baskets. The chosen sister was taught to read, to embroider, and to dwell indoors; if she went out it was only under escort, and with her face buried in a hood of almost incredible size, affording only a glimpse of the poor pale cheeks, so unlike the rosy vigor of the damsels on the mountain-side. The girls, I was told, did not covet this privilege of seclusion; but let us be genteel, or die.

Now all that is left of the Invisible Lady among ourselves is only the remnant of this absurd tradition. In the seaside town where I write, ladies usually go veiled in the streets, and so general is the practice that little girls often veil their dolls. They all suppose it to be done for complexion or for ornament; just as people still hang straps on the backs of their carriages, not knowing that it is a relic of the days when footmen stood there and held on. But the veil represents a tradition of seclusion, whether we know it or not; and the dread of hearing a woman speak in public, or of seeing a woman vote, represents precisely the same tradition. It is entitled to no less respect, and no more.

Like all traditions, it finds something in human nature to which to attach itself. Early girlhood, like early boyhood, needs to be guarded and sheltered, that it may mature unharmed. It is monstrous to make this an excuse for keeping a woman, any more than a man, in a condition of perpetual subordination and seclusion. The young lover wishes to lock up his angel in a little world of her own, where none may intrude. The harem and the seraglio are simply the embodiment of this desire. But the maturer man, and the maturer race, have found that the beloved being should be something more.

After this discovery is made, the theory of the Invisible Lady disappears. It is less of a shock to an American to hear a woman speak in public than it is to an Oriental to see her show her face in public at all. Once open the door of the harem, and she has the freedom of the house: the house includes the front door, and the street is but a prolonged doorstep. With the freedom of the street comes inevitably a free access to the platform, the tribunal, and the pulpit. You might as well try to stop the air in its escape from a punctured balloon, as to try, when woman is once out of the harem, to put her back there. Ceasing to be an Invisible Lady, she must become a visible force: there is no middle ground. There is no danger that she will not be anchored to the cradle, when cradle there is; but it will be by an elastic cable, that will leave her as free to think and vote as to pray. No woman is less a mother because she cares for all the concerns of the world into which her child is born. It was John Quincy Adams who said, defending the political petitions of the women of Plymouth, that "women are not only justified, but exhibit the most exalted virtue, when they do depart from the domestic circle, and enter on the concerns of their country, of humanity, and of their God."

XII.
SACRED OBSCURITY.

In the preface to that ill-named but delightful book, the "Remains of the late Mrs. Richard Trench," there is a singular remark by the editor, her son. He says that "the adage is certainly true in regard to the British matron, *Bene vixit quæ bene latuit*," the meaning of this adage being, "She has lived well who has kept herself well out of sight." Applying this to his beloved mother, he further expresses a regret at disturbing her "sacred obscurity." Then he goes on to disturb it pretty effectually by printing a thick octavo volume of her most private letters.

It is a great source of strength and advantage to reformers, that there are always men preserved to be living examples of this good old Oriental doctrine of "sacred obscurity." Just as Mr. Darwin needs for the demonstration of his theory that the lower orders of creation should still be present in visible form for purposes of comparison, so every reformer needs to fortify his position by showing examples of the original attitude from which society has been gradually emerging. If there had been no Oriental seclusion, many things in the present position of woman would be inexplicable. But when we point to that; when we show that even in the more enlightened Eastern countries it is still held indecorous to allude to the feminine members of a man's family; when we see among the Christian nations of Southern Europe many lingering traits of this same habit of seclusion; and when we find an archdeacon of the English Church still clinging to the theory, even while exhibiting his mother's family letters to the whole world,—we more easily understand the course of development.

These re-assertions of the Oriental theory are simply reversions, as a naturalist would say, to the original type. They are instances of "atavism," like the occasional appearance of six fingers on one hand in a family where the great-great-grandfather happened to possess that ornament. Such instances can always be found, when one takes the pains to look for them. Thus a critic, discussing in the Atlantic Monthly Mr. Mahaffy's book on "Social Life in Greece," is surprised that this writer should quote, in proof of the degradation of woman in Athens, the remark attributed to Pericles, "That woman is best who is least spoken of among men, whether for good or for evil." "In our opinion," adds the reviewer, "that remark was wise then, and is wise now." The Oriental theory is not then, it seems, extinct; and we are spared the pains of proving that it ever existed.

If this theory be true, how falsely has the admiration of mankind been given! If the most obscure woman is best, the most conspicuous must undoubtedly be worst. Tried by this standard, how unworthy must have been Elizabeth Barrett Browning, how reprehensible must be Dorothea Dix, what a model of all that is discreditable is Rosa Bonheur, what a crowning instance of human depravity is Florence Nightingale! Yet how consoling the thought, that, while these disreputable persons were thus wasting their substance in the riotous performance of what the world weakly styled good deeds, there were always women who saw the folly of such efforts, women who by steady devotion to eating, drinking, and sleeping continued to keep themselves in sacred obscurity, and to prove themselves the ornaments of their sex, inasmuch as no human being ever had occasion to mention their names!

But alas for human inconsistency! As for this inverse-ratio theory,—this theory of virtue so exalted that it has never been known or felt or mentioned among men,—it is to be observed that those who hold it are the first to desert it when stirred by an immediate occasion. Just as a slaveholder, in the old times, after demonstrating to you that freedom was a curse to the negro, would instantly turn round, and inflict this greatest of all curses on some slave who had saved his life; so, I fear, would one of these philosophers, if he were profoundly impressed with any great action done by a woman, give the lie to all his theories, and celebrate her fame. In spite of all his fine principles, if he happened to be rescued from drowning by Grace Darling, he would put her name in the newspaper; if he were tended in hospital by Clara Barton, he would sound her praise; and, if his mother wrote as good letters as did Mrs. Trench, he would probably print them to the extent of five hundred pages, as the archdeacon did, and all his gospel of silence would exhale itself in a single sigh of regret in the preface.

XIII.
"OUR TRIALS."

A Providence (R.I.) newspaper remarked some time since that Mrs. Livermore had just delivered in Newport her celebrated lecture, "What shall we do with our Trials?" It was, I suppose, one of those felicitous misprints, by which compositors build better than they know. The real title of the lecture was, "What shall we do with our Girls?" Perhaps it was the unconscious witticism of some poetic young typesetter, to whom damsels were as yet only pleasing pains; or of some premature cynic of the printing-office, who was in the habit of regarding himself as a Blighted Being.

Yet to how many is this morose phrase "humanly adaptive," as Mrs. Browning abstrusely says! Anxious mothers, for instance, will accept it, the mothers of the thousands of surplus maidens—or whatever the statistics say—in Massachusetts. Frederica Bremer inserts in one of her novels an "Extra Leaf on Daughter-full Houses;" an extra that should have a large circulation in many towns of New England. The most heroic and unflinching remedy for this class of trials, so far as my knowledge goes, was that announced by a small relative of my own, aged three, who sitting on the floor thus soliloquized to her doll: "If I had too many daughters, I'd take 'em into the woods and lose 'em—I'd take 'em to the sea and push 'em in: I wouldn't have too many daughters!" She is now a happy wife and mother; but Fate, warned in time by such exceeding plainness of speech, has judiciously endowed her chiefly with sons.

Most of the serious assertion that women are trials comes from masculine wisdom. One hears a good deal of it in summer, at the seaside, from the marriageable youth of some of our chief cities. After a languid hour's chat upon tailors or boots or the proper appointments of a harness,—or of the groom, so perfectly costumed that he seems but a part of the harness,—how often they fall to lamenting the extravagance, the exactions, the general unmarriageableness, of the young women of the present day! Some wit once said that the Pilgrim Mothers had much more to bear than the Pilgrim Fathers, since the Mothers had not only to endure the cold and the hunger, but to endure the Fathers beside. In hearing these remarks I have sometimes thought that these young ladies must be extravagant indeed, if, in addition to their own expenses, they take to themselves so very costly a luxury as a fashionable husband.

And I think that wiser critics than these youths are sometimes tempted into treating these lovely and lovable "trials" in too severely hopeless a way. There is folly enough on the surface, no doubt, and something of it below the surface: yet who does not remember how, in time of need, all these follies proved themselves, during our civil war, but superficial things? The very maidens over whom we had shaken our anxious heads were suddenly those who with pale cheeks bade their lovers leave them, or who changed their gorgeous array for the plain garments of the hospital. So far as I can judge, there is not a young girl within the range of my knowledge who can confidently be insured against marrying a poor artist or a poorer army officer to-morrow, should she once fall thoroughly in love. And, once married, she will very probably develop a power of self-denial, of economy, and of dressing herself and baby gracefully out of the cast-off clothes of her genteel relations,—in a way to put her critics to shame. I think we ought all patiently to endure "trials" that turn to such blessings in the end.

For one, I can truly say, with charming Mrs. Trench in her letters written in 1816, "I do believe the girls of the present day have not lost the power of blushing; and, though I have no grown-up daughters, I enjoy the friendship of some who might be my daughters, in whom the greatest delicacy and modesty are united with perfect ease of manner, and habitual intercourse with the world." And if this is the case,—and I think we shall all own it to be so,—we may as well have the typographical error corrected, after all, and hereafter say—for "trials" read "girls."

XIV.
VIRTUES IN COMMON.

A young friend of mine, who was educated at one of the very best schools for girls in New York City, told me that one day her teacher requested the older girls to write out a list of virtues suitable to manly character, which they did. A month or more later, when this occurrence was well forgotten, the same teacher bade them write out a list of womanly virtues, she making no reference to the other list. Then she made each girl compare her lists; and they all found with surprise that there was no substantial difference between them. The only variation, in most cases, was, that they had put in a rather vague special virtue of "manliness" in the one case, and "womanliness" in the other; a sort of miscellaneous department or "odd drawer," apparently, in which to group all traits not easily analyzed.

The moral is, that, as tested by the common-sense of these young people, duty is duty, and the difference between ethics for men and ethics for women lies simply in practical applications, not in principles.

Who can deny that the philosopher Antisthenes was right when he said, "The virtues of the man and the woman are the same"? Not the Christian, certainly; for he accepts as his highest standard the being who in all history best united the highest qualities of both sexes. Not the metaphysician; for his analysis deals with the human mind as such, not with the mind of either sex. Not the evolutionist; for he is accustomed to trace back qualities to their source, and cannot deny that there is in each sex at least a "survival" of every good and every bad trait. We may say that these qualities are, or may be, or ought to be, distributed unequally between the sexes; but we cannot reasonably deny that each sex possesses a share of every quality, and that what is good in one sex is also good in the other. Man may be the braver, and yet courage in a woman may be nobler than cowardice. Woman may be the purer, and yet purity may be noble in a man.

So clear is this, that some of the very coarsest writers in all literature, and those who have been severest upon women, have yet been obliged to acknowledge it. Take, for instance, Dean Swift, who writes:—

"I am ignorant of any one quality that is amiable in a woman, which is not equally so in a man. I do not except even modesty and gentleness of nature; nor do I know one vice or folly which is not equally detestable in both."

Mrs. Jameson, in her delightful "Commonplace Book," illustrates this admirably by one or two test cases. She takes, for instance, from one of Humboldt's letters a much-admired passage on manly character:—

> "Masculine independence of mind I hold to be in reality the first requisite for the formation of a character of real manly worth. The man who allows himself to be deceived and carried away by his own weakness, may be a very amiable person in other respects, but cannot be called a good man: such beings should not find favor in the eyes of a woman, for a truly beautiful and purely feminine nature should be attracted only by what is highest and noblest in the character of man."

"Take now this same bit of moral philosophy," she says, "and apply it to the feminine character, and it reads quite as well:—

> "'Feminine independence of mind I hold to be in reality the first requisite for the formation of a character of real feminine worth. The woman who allows herself to be deceived and carried away by her own weakness, may be a very amiable person in other respects, but cannot be called a good woman; such beings should not find favor in the eyes of a man, for a truly beautiful and purely manly nature should be attracted only by what is highest and noblest in the character of woman.'"

I have never been able to perceive that there was a quality or grace of character which really belonged exclusively to either sex, or which failed to win honor when wisely exercised by either. It is not thought necessary to have separate editions of books on ethical science, the one for man, the other for woman, like almanacs calculated for different latitudes. The books that vary are not the scientific works, but little manuals of practical application,—"Duties of Men," "Duties of Women." These vary with times and places: where women do not know how to read, no advice on reading will be found in the women's manuals; where it is held wrong for women to uncover the face, it will be laid down in these manuals as a sin. But ethics are ethics: the great principles of morals, as proclaimed either by science or by religion, do not fluctuate for sex; their basis is in the very foundations of right itself.

This grows clearer when we remember that it is equally true in mental science. There is not one logic for men, and another for women; a separate syllogism, a separate induction: the moment we begin to state intellectual principles, that moment we go beyond sex. We deal then with absolute truth. If an observation is wrong, if a process of reasoning is bad, it makes no difference who brings it forward. Any list of mental processes, any inventory of the contents of the mind, would be identical, so far as sex goes, whether compiled by a woman or a man. These things, like the circulation of the blood or the digestion of food, belong clearly to the ground held in common. The London Spectator well said lately,—

"After all, knowledge is knowledge; and there is no more a specifically feminine way of describing correctly the origin of the Lollard movement, or the character of Spenser's poetry, than there is a specifically feminine way of solving a quadratic equation, or of proving the forty-seventh problem of Euclid's first book."

All we can say in modification of this is, that there is, after all, a foundation for the rather vague item of "manliness" and "womanliness" in these schoolgirl lists of duties. There is a difference, after all is said and done; but it is something that eludes analysis, like the differing perfume of two flowers of the same genus and even of the same species. The method of thought must be essentially the same in both sexes; and yet an average woman will put more flavor of something we call instinct into her mental action, and the average man something more of what we call logic into his. Whipple tells us that not a man guessed the plot of Dickens's "Great Expectations," while many women did; and this certainly indicates some average difference of quality or method. So the average opinions of a hundred women, on some question of ethics, might very probably differ from the average of a hundred men, while yet it remains true that "the virtues of the man and the woman are the same."

XV.
INDIVIDUAL DIFFERENCES.

Blackburn, in his entertaining book, "Artists and Arabs," draws a contrast between Frith's painting of the "Derby Day" and Rosa Bonheur's "Horse Fair,"—"the former pleasing the eye by its cleverness and prettiness, the latter impressing the spectator by its power and its truthful rendering of animal life. The difference between the two painters is probably more one of education than of natural gifts. But, whilst the style of the former is grafted on a fashion, the latter is founded on a rock,—the result of a close study of nature, chastened by classic feeling and a remembrance, it may be, of the friezes of the Parthenon."

Now, it is to be observed that this description runs precisely counter to the popular impression as to the work of the two sexes. Novelists like Charles Reade, for instance, who have apparently seen precisely one woman in their lives, and hardly more than one man, and who keep on sketching these two figures most felicitously and brilliantly thenceforward, would be apt to assign these qualities of the artist very differently. Their typical man would do the truthful and powerful work, and everybody would say, "How manly!" Their woman would please by cleverness and prettiness, and everybody would say, "How womanly!" Yet Blackburn shows us that these qualities are individual, not sexual; that they result from temperament, or, he thinks, still more from training. If Rosa Bonheur does better work than Frith, it is not because she is a woman, nor is it in spite of that; but because, setting sex aside, she is a better artist.

This is not denying the distinctions of sex, but only asserting that they are not so exclusive and all-absorbing as is supposed. It is easy to name other grounds of difference which entirely ignore those of sex, striking directly across them, and rendering a different classification necessary. It is thus with distinctions of race or color, for instance. An Indian man and woman are at many points more like to one another than is either to a white person of the same sex. A black-haired man and woman, or a fair-haired man and woman, are to be classified together in these physiological aspects. So of differences of genius: a man and woman of musical temperament and training have more in common than has either with a person who is of the same sex, but who cannot tell one note from another. So two persons of ardent or imaginative temperament are thus far alike, though the gulf of sex divides them; and so are two persons of cold or prosaic temperament. In a mixed school the teacher cannot class together intellectually the boys as such, and the girls as such: bright boys take hold of a lesson very much as bright girls do, and slow girls like slow boys. Nature is too rich, too full, too varied, to be content with a single basis of classification: she has a hundred systems of grouping, according to sex, age, race, temperament, training, and so on; and we get but a narrow view of life when we limit our theories to one set of distinctions.

As a matter of social philosophy, this train of thought logically leads to co-education, impartial suffrage, and free co-operation in all the affairs of life. As a matter of individual duty, it teaches the old moral to "act well your part." No wise person will ever trouble himself or herself much about the limitations of sex in intellectual labor. Rosa Bonheur was not trying to work like a woman, or like a man, or unlike either, but to do her work thoroughly and well. He or she who works in this spirit works nobly, and gives an example which will pass beyond the bounds of sex, and help all. The Abbé Liszt, the most gifted of living pianists, told a friend of mine, his pupil, that he had learned more of music from hearing Madame Malibran sing, than from any thing else whatever.

XVI.
ANGELIC SUPERIORITY.

It is better not to base any plea for woman on the ground of her angelic superiority. The argument proves too much. If she is already so perfect, there is every inducement to let well alone. It suggests the expediency of conforming man's condition to hers, instead of conforming hers to man's. If she is a winged creature, and man can only crawl, it is his condition that needs mending.

Besides, one may well be a little incredulous of these vast claims. Granting some average advantage to woman, it is not of such completeness as to base much argument upon it. The minister looking on his congregation, rarely sees an unmixed angel, either at the head or at the foot of any pew. The domestic servant rarely has the felicity of waiting on an absolute saint at either end of the dinner-table. The lady's-maid has to compare her little observations of human infirmity with those of the valet-de-chambre. The lover worships the beloved, whether man or woman; but marriage bears rather hard on the ideal in either case. And those who pray out of the same book, "Have mercy upon us, miserable sinners," are not supposed to be offering up petitions for each other only.

We all know many women whose lives are made wretched by the sins and follies of their husbands. There are also many men whose lives are turned to long wretchedness by the selfishness, the worldliness, or the bad temper of their wives. Domestic tyranny belongs to neither sex by monopoly. If man tortures or depresses woman, she also has a fearful power to corrupt and deprave man. On the other hand, to quote old Antisthenes once more, "the virtues of the man and woman are the same." A refined man is more refined than a coarse woman. A child-loving man is infinitely tenderer and sweeter toward children than a hard and unsympathetic woman. The very qualities that are claimed as distinctively feminine are possessed more abundantly by many men than by many of what is called the softer sex.

Why is it necessary to say all this? Because there is always danger that we who believe in the equality of the sexes should be led into over-statements, which will re-act against ourselves. It is not safe to say that the ballot-box would be reformed if intrusted to feminine votes alone. Had the voters of the South been all women, it would have plunged earlier into the gulf of secession, dived deeper, and come up even more reluctantly. Were the women of Spain to rule its destinies unchecked, the Pope would be its master, and the Inquisition might be re-established. For all that we can see, the rule of women alone would be as bad as the rule of men alone. It would be as unsafe to give woman the absolute control of man as to make man the master of woman.

Let us be a shade more cautious in our reasonings. Woman needs equal rights, not because she is man's better half, but because she is his other half. She needs them, not as an angel, but as a fraction of humanity. Her political education will not merely help man, but it will help herself. She will sometimes be right in her opinions, and sometimes be altogether wrong; but she will learn, as man learns, by her own blunders. The demand in her behalf is, that she shall have the opportunity to make mistakes, since it is by that means she must become wise.

In all our towns, there is a tendency toward "mixed schools." We rarely hear of the sexes being separated in a school after being once united; but we constantly hear of their being brought together after separation. This is commonly, but mistakenly, recommended as an advantage to the boys alone. I once heard an accomplished teacher remonstrate against this change, when thus urged. "Why should my girls be sacrificed," she said, "to improve your boys?" Six months after, she had learned by experience. "Why," she asked, "did you rest the argument on so narrow a ground? Since my school consisted half of boys, I find with surprise that the change has improved both sexes. My girls are more ambitious, more obedient, and more ladylike. I shall never distrust the policy of mixed schools again."

What is true of the school is true of the family and of the state. It is not good for man, or for woman, to be alone. Granting the woman to be, on the whole, the more spiritually minded, it is still true that each sex needs the other. When the rivet falls from a pair of scissors, we do not have them mended because either half can claim angelic superiority over the other half, but because it takes two halves to make a whole.

XVII.
VICARIOUS HONORS.

There is a story in circulation—possibly without authority—to the effect that a certain young lady has ascended so many Alps that she would have been chosen a member of the English Alpine Club, but for her misfortune in respect to sex. As a matter of personal recognition, however, and, as it were, of approximate courtesy, her dog, who has accompanied her in all her trips, and is not debased by sex, has been elected into the club. She has therefore an opportunity for exercising in behalf of her dog that beautiful self-abnegation which is said to be a part of woman's nature, impelling her always to prefer that her laurels should be worn by somebody else.

The dog probably made no objection to these vicarious honors; nor is any objection made by the young gentlemen who reply eloquently to the toast, "The Ladies" at public dinners, or who kindly consent to be educated at masculine colleges on "scholarships" founded by women. At Harvard University alone there are ten such scholarships,—their income amounting annually to $2,340 in all. Those who receive the emoluments of these funds must reflect within themselves, occasionally, how grand a thing is this power of substitution given to women, and how pleasant are its occasional results to the substitute. It is doubtless more blessed to give than to receive, but to receive without giving has also its pleasures. Very likely the holder of the scholarship, and the orator who rises with his hand on his heart to "reply in behalf of the ladies," may do their appointed work well; and so did the Alpine dog. Yet, after all, but for the work done by his mistress, he would have won no more honor from the Alpine Club than if he had been a chamois.

Nothing since Artemus Ward and his wife's relations has been finer than the generous way in which fathers and brothers disclaim all desire for profits or honors on the part of their feminine relatives. In a certain system of schools once known to me, the boys had prizes of money on certain occasions, but the successful girls at those times received simply a testimonial of honor for each; "the committee being convinced," it was said, "that this was more consonant with the true delicacy and generosity of woman's nature." So in the new arrangements for opening the University of Copenhagen to young women, Karl Blind writes to the New York Evening

Post, that it is expressly provided that they shall not "share in the academic benefices and stipends which have been set apart for male students." Half of these charities may, for aught that appears, have been established originally by women, like the ten Harvard scholarships already named. Women, however, can avail themselves of them only by deputy, as the Alp-climbing young lady is represented by her dog.

It is all a beautiful tribute to the disinterestedness of woman. The only pity is that this virtue, so much admired, should not be reciprocated by showing the like disinterestedness toward her. It does not appear that the butchers and bakers of Copenhagen propose to reduce in the case of women students "the benefices and stipends" which are to be paid for daily food. Young ladies at the university are only prohibited from receiving money, not from needing it. Nor will any of the necessary fatigues of Alpine climbing be relaxed for any young lady because she is a woman. The fatigues will remain in full force, though the laurels be denied. The mountain-passes will make small account of the "tenderness and delicacy of her sex." When the toil is over she will be regarded as too delicate to be thanked for it; but, by way of compensation, the Alpine Club will allow her to be represented by her dog.

XVIII.
THE GOSPEL OF HUMILIATION.

"The silliest man who ever lived," wrote Fanny Fern once, "has always known enough, when he says his prayers, to thank God he was not born a woman." President —— of —— College is not a silly man at all, and he is devoting his life to the education of women; yet he seems to feel as vividly conscious of his superior position as even Fanny Fern could wish. If he had been born a Jew, he would have thanked God, in the appointed ritual, for not having made him a woman. If he had been a Mohammedan, he would have accepted the rule which forbids "a fool, a madman, or a woman" to summon the faithful to prayer. Being a Christian clergyman, with several hundred immortal souls, clothed in female bodies, under his charge, he thinks it his duty, at proper intervals, to notify his young ladies, that, though they may share with men the glory of being sophomores, they still are in a position, as regards the other sex, of hopeless subordination. This is the climax of his discourse, which in its earlier portions contains many good and truthful things:—

> "And, as the woman is different from the man, so is she relative to him. This is true on the other side also. They are bound together by mutual relationship so intimate and vital that the existence of neither is absolutely complete except with reference to the other. But there is this difference, that the relation of woman is, characteristically, that of subordination and dependence. This does not imply inferiority of character, of capacity, of value, in the sight of God or man; and it has been the glory of woman to have accepted the position of formal inferiority assigned her by the Creator, with all its responsibilities, its trials, its possible outward humiliations and sufferings, in the proud consciousness that it is not incompatible with an essential superiority; that it does not prevent her from occupying, if she will, an inward elevation of character, from which she may look down with pitying and helpful love on him she calls her lord. Jesus said, 'Ye know that the princes of the Gentiles exercise dominion over them, and they that are great exercise authority upon them. But it shall not be so among you; but whosoever will be great among you, let him be your minister; and whosoever will be chief among you, let him be your servant, even as the Son of man came, not to be ministered unto, but to minister, and to give his life a ransom for many.' Surely woman need not hesitate to estimate her status by a criterion of dignity sustained by such authority. She need not shrink from a position which was sought by the Son of God, and in whose trials and griefs she will have his sympathy and companionship."

There is a comforting aspect to this discourse, after all. It holds out the hope, that a particularly noble woman may not be personally inferior to a remarkably bad husband, but "may look down with pitying and helpful love on him she calls her lord." The drawback is not merely that it insults woman by a reassertion of a merely historical inferiority, which is steadily diminishing, but that it fortifies this by precisely the same talk about the dignity of subordination which has been used to buttress every oppression since the world began. Never yet was there a pious slaveholder who did not quote to his slaves, on Sunday, precisely the same texts with which President —— favors his meek young pupils. Never yet was there a slaveholder who would not shoot through the head, if he had courage enough, anybody who should attempt to place him in that beautiful position of subjection whose spiritual merits he had been proclaiming. When it came to that, he was like Thoreau, who believed resignation to be a virtue, but preferred "not to practise it unless it was quite necessary."

Thus, when the Rev. Charles C. Jones of Savannah used to address the slaves on their condition, he proclaimed the beauty of obedience in a way to bring tears to their eyes. And this, he frankly assures the masters, is the way to check insurrection and advance their own "pecuniary interests." He says of the slave, that under proper religious instruction "his conscience is enlightened and his soul is awed; ... to God he commits the ordering of his lot, and in his station renders to all their dues, obedience to whom obedience, and honor to whom honor. *He dares not wrest from God his own care and protection.* While he sees a preference in the various conditions of men, he remembers the words of the apostle: 'Art thou called being a servant? Care not for it; but, if thou mayst be free, use it rather. For he that is called in the Lord, being a servant, is the Lord's freeman; likewise, also, he that is called being free, is Christ's servant.'"[4]

[4]. Religious Instruction of the Negroes. Savannah, 1842, pp. 208–211.

I must say that the Rev. Mr. Jones's preaching seems to me precisely as good as Dr. ——'s, and that a sensible woman ought to be as much influenced by the one as was Frederick Douglass by the other—that is, not at all. Let the preacher try "subordination" himself, and see how he likes it. The beauty of service, such as Jesus praised, lay in the willingness of the service: a service that is serfdom loses all beauty, whether rendered by man or by woman. My objection to separate schools and colleges for women is, that they are too apt to end in such instructions as this.

XIX.
"CELERY AND CHERUBS."

There was once a real or imaginary old lady who had got the metaphor of Scylla and Charybdis a little confused. Wishing to describe a perplexing situation, this lady said,—

"You see, my dear, she was between Celery on one side and Cherubs on the other! You know about Celery and Cherubs, don't you? They was two rocks somewhere; and if you didn't hit one, you was pretty sure to run smack on the other."

This describes, as a clever writer in the New York Tribune declares, the present condition of women who "agitate." Their Celery and Cherubs are tears and temper.

It is a good hit, and we may well make a note of it. It is the danger of all reformers, that they will vibrate between discouragement and anger. When things go wrong, what is it one's impulse to do? To be cast down, or to be stirred up; to wring one's hands, or clench one's fists,—in short, tears or temper.

"Mother," said a resolute little girl of my acquaintance, "if the dinner was all spoiled, I wouldn't sit down, and cry! I'd say, 'Hang it!'" This cherub preferred the alternative of temper, on days when the celery turned out badly. Probably her mother was addicted to the other practice, and exhibited the tears.

But as this alternative is found to exist for both sexes, and on all occasions, why charge it especially on the woman-suffrage movement? Men are certainly as much given to ill temper as women; and, if they are less inclined to tears, they make it up in sulks, which are just as bad. Nicholas Nickleby, when the pump was frozen, was advised by Mr. Squeers to "content himself with a dry polish;" and so there is a kind of dry despair into which men fall, which is quite as forlorn as any tears of women. How many a man has doubtless wished at such times that the pump of his lachrymal glands could only thaw out, and he could give his emotions something more than a "dry polish"! The unspeakable comfort some women feel in sitting for ten minutes with a handkerchief over their eyes!

The freshness, the heartiness, the new life visible in them, when the crying is done, and the handkerchief comes down again!

And, indeed, this simple statement brings us to the real truth, which should have been more clearly seen by the writer who tells this story. She is wrong in saying, "It is urged that men and women stand on an equality, are exactly alike." Many of us urge the "equality:" very few of us urge the "exactly alike." An apple and an orange, a potato and a tomato, a rose and a lily, the Episcopal and the Presbyterian churches, Oxford and Cambridge, Yale and Harvard,—we may surely grant equality in each case, without being so exceedingly foolish as to go on and say that they are exactly alike.

And precisely here is the weak point of the whole case, as presented by this writer. Women give way to tears more readily than men? Granted. Is their sex any the weaker for it? Not a bit. It is simply a difference of temperament: that is all. It involves no inferiority. If you think that this habit necessarily means weakness, wait and see! Who has not seen women break down in tears during some domestic calamity, while the "stronger sex" were calm; and who has not seen those same women, that temporary excitement being over, rise up and dry their eyes, and be thenceforth the support and stay of their households, and perhaps bear up the "stronger sex" as a stream bears up a ship? I said once to an experienced physician, watching such a woman, "That woman is really great."—"Of course she is," he answered: "did you ever see a woman who was not great, when the emergency required?"

Now, will women carry this same quality of temperament into their public career? Doubtless: otherwise they would cease to be women. Will it be betraying confidence if I own that I have seen two of the very bravest women of my acquaintance—women who have swayed great audiences—burst into tears, during a committee-meeting, at a moment of unexpected adversity for "the cause"? How pitiable! our critical observers would have thought. In five minutes that April shower had passed, and those women were as resolute and unconquerable as Queen Elizabeth: they were again the natural leaders of those around them; and the cool and tearless men who sat beside them were nothing—men were "a lost art," as some one says—compared with the inexhaustible moral vitality of those two women.

No: the dangers of "Celery and Cherubs" are exaggerated. For temper, women are as good as men, and no better. As for tears, long may they flow!

They are symbols of that mighty distinction of sex which is as ineffaceable and as essential as the difference between land and sea.

XX.
THE NEED OF CAVALRY.

In the interesting Buddhist book, "The Wheel of the Law," translated by Henry Alabaster, there is an account of a certain priest who used to bless a great king, saying, "May your majesty have the firmness of a crow, the audacity of a woman, the endurance of a vulture, and the strength of an ant." The priest then told anecdotes illustrating all of these qualities. Who has not known occasions wherein some daring woman has been the Joan of Arc of a perfectly hopeless cause, taken it up where men shrank, carried it through where they had failed, and conquered by weapons which men would never have thought of using, and would have lacked faith to employ even if put into their hands? The wit, the resources, the audacity of women, have been the key to history and the staple of novels, ever since that larger novel called history began to be written.

How is it done? Who knows the secret of their success? All that any man can say is, that the heart enters largely into the magic. Rogers asserts in his "Table-Talk," that often, when doubting how to act in matters of importance, he had received more useful advice from women than from men. "Women have the understanding of the heart," he said, "which is better than that of the head." Then this instinct, that begins from the heart, reaches the heart also, and through that controls the will. "Win hearts," said Lord Burleigh to Queen Elizabeth, "and you have hands and purses;" and the greatest of English sovereigns, in spite of ugliness and rouge, in spite of coarseness and cruelty and bad passions, was adored by the nation that she first made great.

It seems to me that women are a sort of cavalry force in the army of mankind. They are not always to be relied upon for that steady "hammering away," which was Grant's one method; but there is a certain Sheridan quality about them, light-armed, audacious, quick, irresistible. They go before the main army; their swift wits go scouting far in advance; they are the first to scent danger, or to spy out chances of success. Their charge is like that of a Tartar horde, or the wild sweep of the Apaches. They are upon you from some wholly unexpected quarter; and this respectable, systematic, well-drilled masculine force is caught and rolled over and over in the dust, before the man knows what has hit him. But, even if repelled and beaten off, this formidable cavalry is unconquered: routed and in confusion to-day, it comes back upon you to-morrow—fresh, alert, with new devices, bringing new dangers. In dealing with it, as the French complained of the Arabs in Algiers, "Peace is not to be purchased by victory." And, even if all seems lost, with what a brilliant final charge it will cover a retreat!

Decidedly, we need cavalry. In older countries, where it has been a merely undisciplined and irregular force, it has often done mischief; and public men, from Demosthenes down, have been lamenting that measures which the statesman has meditated a whole year, may be overturned in a day by a woman. Under our American government we have foolishly attempted to leave out this arm of the service altogether; and much of the alleged dulness of our American history has come from this attempt. Those who have been trained in the various reforms where woman has taken an equal part—the anti-slavery reform especially—know well how much of the energy, the dash, the daring, of those movements, have come from her. A revolution with a woman in it is stronger than the established order that omits her. It is not that she is superior to man, but she is different from man; and we can no more spare her than we could spare the cavalry from an army.

XXI.
"THE REASON FIRM, THE TEMPERATE WILL."

It is a part of the necessary theory of republican government, that every class and race shall be judged by its highest types, not its lowest. The proposition of the French revolutionary statesman, to begin the work of purifying the world by arresting all the cowards and knaves, is liable to the objection that it would find victims in every circle. Republican government begins at the other end, and assumes that the community generally has good intentions at least, and some common sense, however it may be with individuals. Take the very quality which the newspapers so often deny to women,—the quality of steadiness. "In fact, men's great objection to the entrance of the female mind into politics is drawn from a suspicion of its unsteadiness on matters in which the feelings could by any possibility be enlisted." Thus says the New York Nation. Let us consider this implied charge against women, and consider it not by generalizing from a single instance,—"just like a woman," as the editors would doubtless say, if a woman had done it,—but by observing whole classes of that sex, taken together.

These classes need some care in selection, for the plain reason that there are comparatively few circles in which women have yet been allowed enough freedom of scope, or have acted sufficiently on the same plane with men, to furnish a fair estimate of their probable action, were they enfranchised. Still there occur to me three such classes,—the anti-slavery women, the Quaker women, and the women who conduct philanthropic operations in our large cities. If the alleged unsteadiness of women is to be felt in public affairs, it would have been felt in these organizations. Has it been so felt?

Of the anti-slavery movement I can personally testify,—and I have heard the same point fully recognized among my elders, such as Garrison, Phillips, and Quincy,—that the women contributed their full share, if not more than their share, to the steadiness of that movement, even in times when the feelings were most excited, as, for instance, in fugitive-slave cases. Who that has seen mobs practically put down, and mayors cowed into decency, by the silent dignity of those rows of women who sat, with their knitting, more imperturbable than the men, can read without a smile these doubts of the "steadiness" of that sex? Again, among Quaker women, I have asked the opinion of prominent Friends, as of John G. Whittier, whether it has been the experience of that body that women were more flighty and unsteady than men in their official action; and have been uniformly answered in the negative. And finally, as to benevolent organizations, a good test is given in the fact,—first pointed out, I believe, by that eminently practical philanthropist, Rev. Augustus Woodbury of Providence,—that the whole tendency has been, during the last twenty years, to put the management, even the financial control, of our benevolent societies, more and more into the hands of women, and that there has never been the slightest reason to reverse this policy. Ask the secretaries of the various boards of State Charities, or the officers of the Social Science Associations, if they have found reason to complain of the want of steadfast qualities in the "weaker sex." Why is it that the legislation of Massachusetts has assigned the class requiring the steadiest of all supervision—the imprisoned convicts—to "five commissioners of prisons, two of whom shall be women"? These are the points which it would be worthy of our journals to consider, instead of hastily generalizing from single instances. Let us appeal from the typical woman of the editorial picture,—fickle, unsteady, foolish,—to the nobler conception of womanhood which the poet Wordsworth found fulfilled in his own household:—

> "A being breathing thoughtful breath,
> A traveller betwixt life and death;
> *The reason firm, the temperate will;*
> *Endurance, foresight, strength and skill*;
> A perfect woman, nobly planned
> To warn, to comfort, to command,
> And yet a spirit still, and bright
> With something of an angel light."

XXII.
"ALLURES TO BRIGHTER WORLDS, AND LEADS THE WAY."

When the Massachusetts House of Representatives had "School Suffrage" under consideration, the other day, the suggestion was made by one of the pithiest and quaintest of the speakers, that men were always better for the society of women, and therefore ought to vote in their company. "If all of us," he said, "would stay away from all places where we cannot take our wives and daughters with us, we should keep better company than we now do." This expresses a feeling which grows more and more common among the better class of men, and which is the key to much progress in the condition of women. There can be no doubt that the increased association of the sexes in society, in school, in literature, tends to purify these several spheres of action. Yet, when we come to philosophize on this, there occur some perplexities on the way.

For instance, the exclusion of woman from all these spheres was in ancient Greece almost complete; yet the leading Greek poets, as Homer and the tragedians, are exceedingly chaste in tone, and in this respect beyond most of the great poets of modern nations. Again no European nation has quite so far sequestered and subordinated women as has Spain; and yet the whole tone of Spanish literature is conspicuously grave and decorous. This plainly indicates that race has much to do with the matter, and that the mere admission or exclusion of women is but one among several factors. In short, it is easy to make out a case by a rhetorical use of the facts on one side; but, if we look at all the facts, the matter presents greater difficulties.

Again, it is to be noted that in several countries the first women who have taken prominent part in literature have been as bad as the men; as, for instance, Marguerite of Navarre and Mrs. Aphra Behn. This might indeed be explained by supposing that they had to gain entrance into literature by accepting the dissolute standards which they found prevailing. But it would probably be more correct to say that these standards themselves were variable, and that their variation affected, at certain periods, women as well as men. Marguerite of Navarre wrote religious books as well as merry stories; and we know from Lockhart's Life of Scott, that ladies of high character in Edinburgh used to read Mrs. Behn's tales and plays aloud, at one time, with delight,—although one of the same ladies found, in her old age, that she could not read them to herself without blushing. Shakspeare puts coarse repartees into the mouths of women of stainless virtue. George Sand is not considered an unexceptionable writer; but she tells us in her autobiography that she found among her grandmother's papers poems and satires so indecent that she could not read them through, and yet they bore the names of *abbés* and gentlemen whom she remembered in her childhood as models of dignity and honor. Voltaire inscribes to ladies of high rank, who doubtless regarded it as a great compliment, verses such as not even a poet of the English "fleshly school" would now print at all. In "Poems by Eminent Ladies,"—published in 1755 and reprinted in 1774,—there are one or two poems as gross and disgusting as any thing in Swift; yet their authors were thought reputable women. Allan Ramsay's "Tea-Table Miscellany"—a collection of English and Scottish songs—was first published in 1724; and in his preface to the sixteenth edition the editor attributes its great success, especially among the ladies, to the fact that he has carefully excluded all grossness, "that the modest voice and ear of the fair singer might meet with no affront;" and adds, "the chief bent of all my studies being to attain their good graces." There is no doubt of the great popularity enjoyed by the book in all circles; yet it contains a few songs which the most licentious newspaper would not now publish. The inference is irresistible, from this and many other similar facts, that the whole tone of manners and decency has very greatly improved among the European races within a century and a half.

I suspect the truth to be, that, besides the visible influence of race and religion, there has been an insensible and almost unconscious improvement in each sex, with respect to these matters, as time has passed on; and that the mutual desire to please has enabled each sex to help the other,—the sex which is naturally the more refined taking the lead. But I should lay more stress on this mutual influence, and less on mere feminine superiority, than would be laid by many. It is often claimed by teachers that co-education helps not only boys, but also girls, to develop greater propriety of manners. When the sexes are wholly separate, or associate on terms of entire inequality, no such good influence occurs: the more equal the association, the better for both parties. After all, the Divine model is to be found in the family; and the best ingenuity cannot improve much upon it.

THE HOME.

"In respect to the powers and rights of married women, the law is by no means abreast of the spirit of the age. Here are seen the old fossil footprints of feudalism. The law relating to woman tends to make every family a barony or a monarchy or a despotism, of which the husband is the baron, king, or despot, and the wife the dependent, serf, or slave. That this is not always the fact, is not due to the law, but to the enlarged humanity which spurns the narrow limits of its rules. The progress of civilization has changed the family from a barony to a republic; but the law has not kept pace with the advance of ideas, manners, and customs."—W. W. STORY's *Treatise on Contracts not under Seal*, § 84,—third edition, p. 89.

XXIII.
WANTED—HOMES.

We see advertisements, occasionally, of "Homes for Aged Women," and more rarely "Homes for Aged Men." The question sometimes suggests itself, whether it would not be better to begin the provision earlier, and see that homes are also provided, in some form, for the middle-aged and even the young. The trouble is, I suppose, that as it takes two to make a bargain, so it takes at least two to make a home; and unluckily it takes only one to spoil it.

Madame Roland once defined marriage as an institution where one person undertakes to provide happiness for two; and many failures are accounted for, no doubt, by this false basis. Sometimes it is the man, more often the woman, of whom this extravagant demand is made. There are marriages which have proved a wreck almost wholly through the fault of the wife. Nor is this confined to wedded homes alone. I have known a son who lived alone, patiently and uncomplainingly, with that saddest of all conceivable companions, a drunken mother. I have known another young man who supported in his own home a mother and sister, both habitual drunkards. All these were American-born, and all of respectable social position. A home shadowed by such misery is not a home, though it might have been a home but for the sins of women. Such instances are, however, rare and occasional compared with the cases where the same offence in the husband makes ruin of the home.

Then there are the cases where indolence, or selfishness, or vanity, or the love of social excitement, in the woman, unfits her for home life. Here we come upon ground where perhaps woman is the greater sinner. It must be remembered, however, that against this must be balanced the neglect produced by club-life, or by the life of society-membership, in a man. A brilliant young married belle in London once told me that she was glad her husband was so fond of his club, for it amused him every night while she went to balls. "Married men do not go much into society here," she said, "unless they are regular flirts,—which I do not think my husband would ever be, for he is very fond of me,—so he goes every night to his club, and gets home about the same time that I do. It is a very nice arrangement." It was apparently spoken in all the fearlessness of innocence, but I believe that it has since ended in a "separation."

It is common to denounce club-life in our large cities as destructive of the home. The modern club is simply a more refined substitute for the old-fashioned tavern, and is on the whole an advance in morals as well as manners. In our large cities a man in a certain social coterie belongs to a club, if he can afford it, as a means of contact with his fellows, and to have various conveniences which he cannot so economically obtain at home. A few haunt them constantly: the many use them occasionally. More absorbing than clubs, perhaps, are the secret societies which have so revived among us since the war, and which consume time so fearfully. There was a case mentioned in the newspapers lately of a man who belonged to some twenty of these associations; and when he died, and each wished to conduct his funeral, great was the strife! In the small city where I write, there are seventeen secret societies down in the directory, and I suppose as many more not so conspicuous. I meet men who assure me that they habitually attend a societymeeting every evening of the week except Sunday, and a church meeting then. These are rarely men of leisure: they are usually mechanics or business men of some kind, who are hard at work all day, and never see their families except at meal-times. Their case is far worse, so far as absence from home is concerned, than that of the "club-men" of large cities; for these are often men of leisure, who, if married, at least make home one of their lounging-places, which the secret-society men do not.

I honestly believe that this melancholy desertion of the home is largely due to the traditional separation between the alleged spheres of the sexes. The theory still prevails largely, that home is the peculiar province of the woman, that she has almost no duties out of it; and hence, naturally enough, that the husband has almost no duties in it. If he is amused there, let him stay there; but, as it is not his recognized sphere of duty, he is not actually violating any duty by absenting himself. This theory even pervades our manuals of morals, of metaphysics, and of popular science; and it is not every public teacher who has the manliness, having once stated it, to modify his statement, as did the venerable President Hopkins of Williams College, when lecturing the other day to the young ladies of Vassar.

"I would," he said, "at this point correct my teaching in 'The Law of Love' to the effect that home is peculiarly the sphere of woman, and civil government that of man. *I now regard the home as the joint sphere of man and woman, and the sphere of civil government more of an open question as between the two.* It is, however, to be lamented that the present agitation concerning the rights of woman is so much a matter of 'rights' rather than of 'duties,' as the reform of the latter would involve the former."

If our instructors in moral philosophy will only base their theory of ethics as broadly as this, we shall no longer need to advertise "Homes Wanted;" for the joint efforts of men and women will soon provide them.

XXIV.
THE ORIGIN OF CIVILIZATION.

Nothing throws more light on the whole history of woman than the first illustration in Sir John Lubbock's "Origin of Civilization." A young girl, almost naked, is being dragged furiously along the ground by a party of naked savages, armed literally to the teeth, while those of another band grasp her by the arm, and almost tear her asunder in the effort to hold her back. These last are her brothers and her friends; the others are—her enemies? As you please to call them. They are her future husband and his kinsmen, who have come to aid him in his wooing.

This was the primitive rite of marriage. Vestiges of it still remain among savage nations. And all the romance and grace of the most refined modern marriage—the orange-blossoms, the bridal veil, the church service, the wedding-feast—these are only the "bright consummate flower" reared by civilization from that rough seed. All the brutal encounter is softened into this. Nothing remains of the barbarism except the one word "obey," and even that is going.

Now, to say that a thing is going, is to say that it will presently be gone. To say that any thing is changed, is to say that it is to change further. If it never has been altered, perhaps it will not be; but a proved alteration of an inch in a year opens the way to an indefinite modification. The study of the glaciers, for instance, began with the discovery that they had moved; and from that moment no one doubted that they were moving all the time. It is the same with the position of woman. Once open your eyes to the fact that it has changed, and who is to predict where the matter shall end? It is sheer folly to say, "Her relative position will always be what it has been," when one glance at Sir John Lubbock's picture shows that there is no fixed "has been," but that her original position was long since altered and revised. Those who still use this argument are like those who laughed at the lines of stakes which Agassiz planted across the Aar glacier in 1840. But the stakes settled the question, and proved the motion. *Pero si muove*: "But it moves."

The motion once proved, the whole range of possible progress is before us. The amazement of that formerly "heathen Chinee" in Boston, the other day, when he saw a woman addressing a missionary meeting; the astonishment of all English visitors when young ladies hear classes in geometry and Latin, in our high schools; the surprise of foreigners at seeing the rough throng in the Cooper Institute reading-room submit to the sway of one young woman with a crochet-needle—all these simply testify to the fact that the stakes have moved. That they have yet been carried half way to the end, who knows? What a step from the horrible nuptials of those savage days to the poetic marriage of Robert Browning and Elizabeth Barrett—the "Sonnets from the Portuguese" on one side, the "One Word More" on the other! But who can say that the whole relation between man and woman reached its climax there, and that where the past has brought changes so vast the future is to add nothing? Who knows that, when "the world's great bridals come," people may not look back with pity, even on this era of the Brownings? Probably even Elizabeth Barrett promised to obey!

At any rate, it is safe to say that each step concedes the probability of another. Even from the naked barbarian to the veiled Oriental, from the savage hut to the carefully enshrined harem, is a step forward. It is another step in the spiral line of progress to the unveiled face and comparatively free movements of the modern English or American woman. From the kitchen to the public lecture-room, from that to the lecture-platform, and from that again to the ballot-box,—these are far slighter steps than those which have already lifted the savage girl of Sir John Lubbock's picture into the possession of the alphabet and the dignity of a home. So easy are these future changes beside those of the past, that to doubt their possibility is as if Agassiz, after tracing year by year the motion of his Alpine glacier, should deny its power to move one inch farther into the sunny valley, and there to melt harmlessly away.

XXV.
THE LOW-WATER MARK.

We constantly see it assumed, in arguments against any step in the elevation of woman, that her position is a thing fixed permanently by nature, so that there can be in it no great or essential change. Every successive modification is resisted as "a reform against nature;" and this argument from permanence is always that appealing most strongly to conservative minds. Let us see how the facts confirm it.

A story is going the rounds of the newspapers in regard to a Russian peasant and his wife. For some act of disobedience the peasant took the law into his own hands; and his mode of discipline was to tie the poor creature naked to a post in the street, and to call on every passer-by to strike her a blow. Not satisfied with this, he placed her on the ground, and tied heavy weights on her limbs until one arm was broken. When finally released, she made a complaint against him in court. The court discharged him on the ground that he had not exceeded the legal authority of a husband. Encouraged by this, he caused her to be arrested in return; and the same court sentenced her to another public whipping for disobedience.

No authority was given for this story in the newspaper where I saw it; but it certainly did not first appear in a woman-suffrage newspaper, and cannot therefore be a manufactured "outrage." I use it simply to illustrate the low-water mark at which the position of woman may rest, in the largest Christian nation of the world. All the refinements, all the education, all the comparative justice, of modern society, have been gradually upheaved from some such depth as this. When the gypsies described by Leland treat even the ground trodden upon by a woman as impure, they simply illustrate the low plane from which all the elevation of woman has begun. All these things show that the position of that sex in society, so far from being a thing in itself permanent, has been in reality the most variable of all factors in the social problem. And this inevitably suggests the question, Are we any more sure that her present position is finally and absolutely fixed than were those who observed it at any previous time in the world's history? Granting that her condition was once at low-water mark, who is authorized to say that it has yet reached high-tide?

It is very possible that this Russian wife, once scourged back to submission, ended her days in the conviction, and taught to her daughters, that such was a woman's rightful place. When an American woman of to-day says, "I have all the rights I want," is she on any surer ground? Grant that the difference is vast between the two. How do we know that even the later condition is final, or that any thing is final but entire equality before the laws? It is not many years since William Story—in a legal work inspired and revised by his father, the greatest of American jurists—wrote this indignant protest against the injustice of the old common law:—

"In respect to the powers and rights of married women, the law is by no means abreast of the spirit of the age. Here are seen the old fossil footprints of feudalism. The law relating to woman tends to make every family a barony or a monarchy, or a despotism, of which the husband is the baron, king, or despot, and the wife the dependent, serf, or slave. That this is not always the fact, is not due to the law, but to the enlarged humanity which spurns the narrow limits of its rules. The progress of civilization has changed the family from a barony to a republic; but the law has not kept pace with the advance of ideas, manners, and customs. And, although public opinion is a check to legal rules on the subject, the rules are feudal and stern. Yet the position of woman throughout history serves as the criterion of the freedom of the people or an age. When man shall despise that right which is founded only on might, woman will be free and stand on an equal level with him,—a friend and not a dependent."[5]

5. Story's Treatise on the Law of Contracts not under Seal, p. 89, § 84.

We know that the law is greatly changed and ameliorated in many places since Story wrote this statement; but we also know how almost every one of these changes was resisted: and who is authorized to say that the final and equitable fulfilment is yet reached?

XXVI.
"OBEY."

After witnessing the marriage ceremony of the Episcopal Church, the other day, I walked down the aisle with the young rector who had officiated. It was natural to speak of the beauty of the Church service on an occasion like that; but, after doing this, I felt compelled to protest against the unrighteous pledge to obey. "I hope," I said, "to live to see that word expunged from the Episcopal service, as it has been from that of the Methodists."

"Why?" he asked. "Is it because you know that they will not obey, whatever their promise?"

"Because they ought not," I said.

"Well," said he, after a few moments' reflection, and looking up frankly, "I do not think they ought!"

Here was a young clergyman of great earnestness and self-devotion, who included it among the sacred duties of his life to impose upon ignorant young girls a solemn obligation, which he yet thought they ought not to incur, and did not believe that they would keep. There could hardly be a better illustration of the confusion in the public mind, or the manner in which "the subjection of woman" is being outgrown, or the subtile way in which this subjection has been interwoven with sacred ties, and baptized "duty."

The advocates of woman suffrage are constantly reproved for using the terms "subjection," "oppression," and "slavery," as applied to woman. They simply commit the same sin as that committed by the original abolitionists. They are "as harsh as truth, as uncompromising as justice." Of course they talk about oppression and emancipation. It is the word *obey* that constitutes the one, and shows the need of the other. Whoever is pledged to obey is technically and literally a slave, no matter how many roses surround the chains. All the more so if the slavery is self-imposed, and surrounded by all the prescriptions of religion. Make the marriage-tie as close as Church or State can make it; but let it be equal, impartial. That it may be so, the word *obey* must be abandoned or made reciprocal. Where invariable obedience is promised, equality is gone.

That there may be no doubt about the meaning of this word in the marriage-covenant, the usages of nations often add symbolic explanations. These are generally simple and brutal enough to be understood. The Hebrew ceremony, when the bridegroom took off his slipper and struck the bride on the neck as she crossed his threshold, was unmistakable. As my black sergeant said, when a white prisoner questioned his authority, and he pointed to the *chevrons* on his sleeve, "Dat mean guv'ment." All these forms mean simply government also. The ceremony of the slipper has now no recognition, except when people fling an old shoe after the bride, which is held by antiquarians to be the same observance. But it is all preserved and concentrated into a single word, when the bride promises to obey.

The deepest wretchedness that has ever been put into human language, or that has exceeded it, has grown out of that pledge. There is no misery on earth like that of a pure and refined woman who finds herself owned, body and soul, by a drunken, licentious, brutal man. The very fact that she is held to obedience by a spiritual tie makes it worse. Chattel-slavery was not so bad; for, though the master might pervert religion for his own satisfaction, he could not impose upon the slave. Never yet did I see a negro slave who thought it a duty to obey his master; and therefore there was always some dream of release. But who has not heard of some delicate and refined woman, one day of whose torture was equivalent to years of that possible to an obtuser frame,—who had the door of escape ready at hand for years, and yet died a lingering death rather than pass through it; and this because she had promised to obey!

It is said of one of the most gifted women who ever trod American soil, —she being of English birth,—that, before she obtained the divorce which separated her from her profligate husband, she once went for counsel to the wife of her pastor. She unrolled before her the long catalogue of merciless outrages to which she had been subject, endangering finally her health, her life, and that of her children born and to be born. When she turned at last for advice to her confessor, with the agonized inquiry, "What is it my duty to do?"—"Do?" said the stern adviser: "Lie down on the floor, and let your husband trample on you if he will. That is a woman's duty."

The woman who gave this advice was not naturally inhuman nor heartless: she had simply been trained in the school of obedience. The Jesuit doctrine, that a priest should be as a corpse, *perinde ac cadaver*, in the hands of a superior priest, is not worse. Woman has no right to delegate, nor man to assume, a responsibility so awful. Just in proportion as it is consistently carried out, it trains men from boyhood into self-indulgent tyrants; and, while some women are transformed by it to saints, others are crushed into deceitful slaves. That this was the result of chattel-slavery, this nation has at length learned. We learn more slowly the profounder and more subtile moral evil that follows from the unrighteous promise to obey.

XXVII.
WOMAN IN THE CHRYSALIS.

When the bride receives the ring upon her finger, and utters—if she utters it—the unnatural promise to obey, she fancies a poetic beauty in the rite. Turning of her own free will from her maiden liberty, she voluntarily takes the yoke of service upon her. This is her view; but is this the historic fact in regard to marriage? Not at all. The pledge of obedience—the whole theory of inequality in marriage—is simply what is left to us of a former state of society, in which every woman, old or young, must obey somebody. The state of tutelage, implied in such a marriage, is merely what is left of the old theory of the "Perpetual Tutelage of Women," under the Roman law.

Roman law, from which our civil law is derived, has its foundation evidently in patriarchal tradition. It recognized at first the family only, and that family was held together by parental power (*patria potestas*). If the father died, his powers passed to the son or grandson, as the possible head of a new family; but these powers never could pass to a woman, and every woman, of whatever age, must be under somebody's legal control. Her father dying, she was still subject through life to her nearest male relations, or to her father's nominees, as her guardians. She was under perpetual guardianship, both as to person or property. No years, no experience, could make her any thing but a child before the law.

In Oriental countries the system was still more complete. "A man," says the Gentoo Code of Laws, "must keep his wife so much in subjection that she by no means be mistress of her own action. If the wife have her own free will, notwithstanding she be of a superior caste, she will behave amiss." But this authority, which still exists in India, is not merely conjugal. The husband exerts it simply as being the wife's legal guardian. If the woman be unmarried or a widow, she must be as rigorously held under some other guardianship. It is no uncommon thing for a woman in India to be the ward of her own son. Lucretia Mott or Florence Nightingale would there be in personal subjection to somebody. Any man of legal age would be recognized as a fit custodian for them, but there must be a man.

With some variation of details at different periods, the same system prevailed essentially at Rome, down to the time when Rome became

Christian. Those who wish for particulars will find them in an admirable chapter (the fifth) of Maine's "Ancient Law." At one time the husband was held to possess the *patria potestas,* or parental power, in its full force. By law "the woman passed *in manum viri,* that is, she became the daughter of her husband." All she had became his, and after his death she was retained in the same strict tutelage by any guardians his will might appoint. Afterwards, to soften this rigid bond, the woman was regarded in law as being temporarily deposited by her family with her husband; the family appointed guardians over her: and thus, between the two tyrannies, she won a sort of independence. Then came Christianity, and swept away the parental authority for married women, concentrating all upon the husband. Hence our legislation bears the mark of a double origin, and woman is half recognized as an equal and half as a slave.

It is necessary to remember, therefore, that all the relation of subjection in marriage is merely the residue of an unnatural system, of which all else is long since outgrown. It would have seemed to an ancient Roman a matter of course that a woman should, all her life long, obey the guardians set over her person. It still seems to many people a matter of course that she should obey her husband. To others among us, on the contrary, both these theories of obedience seem barbarous, and the one is merely a relic of the other.

We cannot disregard the history of the Theory of Tutelage. If we could believe that a chrysalis is always a chrysalis, and a butterfly always a butterfly, we could easily leave each to its appropriate sphere; but when we see the chrysalis open, and the butterfly come half out of it, we know that sooner or later it must spread wings, and fly. The theory of tutelage is the chrysalis. Woman is the butterfly. Sooner or later she will be wholly out.

XXVIII.
TWO AND TWO.

A young man of very good brains was telling me, the other day, his dreams of his future wife. Rattling on, more in joke than in earnest, he said, "She must be perfectly ignorant, and a bigot: she must know nothing, and believe every thing. I should wish to have her call to me from the adjoining room, 'My dear, what do two and two make?'"

It did not seem to me that his demand would be so very hard to fill, since bigotry and ignorance are to be had almost anywhere for the asking; and, as for two and two, I should say that it had always been the habit of women to ask that question of some man, and to rest easily satisfied with the answer. They have generally called, as my friend wished, from some other room, saying, "My dear, what do two and two make?" and the husband or father or brother has answered and said, "My dear, they make four for a man, and three for a woman."

At any given period in the history of woman, she has adopted man's whim as the measure of her rights; has claimed nothing; has sweetly accepted any thing: the law of two-and-two itself should be at his discretion. At any given moment, so well was his interpretation received, that it stood for absolute right. In Rome a woman, married or single, could not testify in court; in the middle ages, and down to quite modern times, she could not hold real estate; ten years ago she could not, in New England, obtain a collegiate education; even now she cannot vote.

The first principles of republican government are so rehearsed and re-rehearsed, that one would think they must become "as plain as that two and two make four." But we find throughout, that, as Emerson said of another class of reasoners, "Their two is not the real two; their four is not the real four." We find different numerals and diverse arithmetical rules for the two sexes; as, in some Oriental countries, men and women speak different dialects of the same language.

In novels the hero often begins by dreaming, like my friend, of an ideal wife, who shall be ignorant of every thing, and have only brains enough to be bigoted. Instead of sighing, like Falstaff, "Oh for a fine young thief, of the age of two and twenty or thereabouts!" the hero sighs for a fine young idiot of similar age. When the hero is successful in his search and wooing, the novelist sometimes mercifully removes the young woman early, like David Copperfield's Dora, she bequeathing the bereaved husband, on her death-bed, to a woman of sense. In real life these convenient interruptions do not commonly occur, and the foolish youth regrets through many years that he did not select an Agnes instead.

The acute observer Stendhal says,—

"In Paris, the highest praise for a marriageable girl is to say, 'She has great sweetness of character and the disposition of a lamb.' Nothing produces more impression on fools who are looking out for wives. I think I see the interesting couple, two years after, breakfasting together on a dull day, with three tall lackeys waiting upon them!"

And he adds, still speaking in the interest of men,—

"Most men have a period in their career when they might do something great, a period when nothing seems impossible. The ignorance of women spoils for the human race this magnificent opportunity; and love, at the utmost, in these days, only inspires a young man to learn to ride well, or to make a judicious selection of a tailor."[6]

6. De L'Amour, par de Stendhal (Henri Beyle). Paris, 1868 [written in 1822], pp. 182, 198.

Society, however, discovers by degrees that there are conveniences in every woman's knowing the four rules of arithmetic for herself. Two and two come to the same amount on a butcher's bill, whether the order be given by a man or a woman; and it is the same in all affairs or investments, financial or moral. We shall one day learn that with laws, customs, and public affairs it is even so. Once get it rooted in a woman's mind, that, for her, two and two make three only, and sooner or later the accounts of the whole human race fail to balance.

XXIX.
A MODEL HOUSEHOLD.

There is an African bird called the hornbill, whose habits are in some respects a model. The female builds her nest in a hollow tree, lays her eggs, and broods on them. So far, so good. Then the male feels that he must also contribute some service; so he walls up the hole closely, giving only room for the point of the female's bill to protrude. Until the eggs are hatched, she is thenceforth confined to her nest, and is in the mean time fed assiduously by her mate, who devotes himself entirely to this object. Dr. Livingstone has seen these nests in Africa, Layard and others in Asia, and Wallace in Sumatra.

Personally I have never seen a hornbill's nest. The nearest approach I ever made to it was when in Fayal I used to pass near a gloomy mansion, of which the front windows were walled up, and only one high window was visible in the rear, beyond the reach of eyes from any neighboring house. In this cheerful abode, I was assured, a Portuguese lady had been for many years confined by her jealous husband. It was long since any neighbor had caught a glimpse of her, but it was supposed that she was alive. There is no reason to doubt that her husband fed her well. It was simply a case of human hornbill, with the imprisonment made perpetual.

I have more than once asked lawyers whether, in communities where the old common law prevailed, there was any thing to prevent such an imprisonment of a married woman; and they have always answered, "Nothing but public opinion." Where the husband has the legal custody of the wife's person, no *habeas corpus* can avail against him. The hornbill household is based on a strict application of the old common law. A Hindoo household was a hornbill household: "a woman, of whatsoever age, should never be mistress of her own actions," said the code of Menu. An Athenian household was a hornbill's nest, and great was the outcry when some Aspasia broke out of it. When Mrs. Sherman petitions Congress against the emancipation of woman, we seem to hear the twittering of the hornbill mother, imploring to be left inside.

Under some forms, the hornbill theory becomes respectable. There are many peaceful families, innocent though torpid, where the only dream of existence is to have plenty of quiet, plenty of food, and plenty of well-fed children. For them this African household is a sufficient model. The wife is "a home body." The husband is "a good provider." These are honest people, and have a right to speak. The hornbill theory is only dishonest when it comes—as it often comes—from women who lead the life, not of good stay-at-home fowls, but of paroquets and humming-birds,—who sorrowfully bemoan the active habits of enlightened women, while they themselves

> "Bear about the mockery of woe
> To midnight dances and the public show."

It is from these women, in Washington, New York, and elsewhere, that the loudest appeal for the hornbill standard of domesticity proceeds. Put them to the test, and give them their chicken-salad and champagne through a hole in the wall only, and see how they like it.

But even the most honest and peaceful conservatives will one day admit that the hornbill is not the highest model. Plato thought that "the soul of our grandame might haply inhabit the body of a bird;" but Nature has kindly provided various types of bird-households to suit all varieties of taste. The bright orioles, filling the summer boughs with color and with song, are as truly domestic in the freedom of their airy nest as the poor hornbills who ignorantly make home into a dungeon. And certainly each new generation of orioles, spreading their free wings from that pendent cradle, are a happier illustration of judicious nurture than are the uncouth little offspring of the hornbills, whom Wallace describes as "so flabby and semi-transparent as to resemble a bladder of jelly, furnished with head, legs, and rudimentary wings, but with not a sign of a feather, except a few lines of points indicating where they would come."

XXX.
A SAFEGUARD FOR THE FAMILY.

Many German-Americans are warm friends of woman suffrage; but the editors of "Puck," it seems, are not. In a late number of that comic journal, it had an unfavorable cartoon on this reform; and in a following number,— the number, by the way, which contains that amusing illustration of the vast seaside hotels of the future, with the cheering announcement, "Only one mile to the barber's shop," and "Take the cars to the dining-room,"—a lady comes to the rescue, and bravely defends woman suffrage. It seems that the original cartoon depicted in the corner a pretty family scene, representing father, mother, and children seated happily together, with the melancholy motto, "Nevermore, nevermore!" And when the correspondent, Mrs. Blake, very naturally asks what this touching picture has to do with woman suffrage, Puck says, "If the husband in our 'pretty family scene' should propose to vote for the candidate who was obnoxious to his wife, would this 'pretty family scene' continue to be a domestic paradise, or would it remind the spectator of the region in which Dante spent his 'fortnight off'?"

It is beautiful to see how much anxiety there is to preserve the family. Every step in the modification of the old common law, whereby the wife was, in Baron Alderson's phrase, "the servant of her husband," was resisted as tending to endanger the family. That the wife should control her own earnings, so that her husband should not have the right to collect them in order to pay his gambling-debts, was declared by English advocates, in the celebrated case of the Hon. Mrs. Norton, the poetess, to imperil all the future peace of British households. Even the liberal-minded "Punch," about the time Girton College was founded in England, expressed grave doubts whether the harmony of wedded unions would not receive a blow, from the time when wives should be liable to know more Greek than their husbands. Yet the marriage relation has withstood these innovations. It has not been impaired, either by separate rights, private earnings, or independent Greek: can it be possible that a little voting will overthrow it?

The very ground on which woman suffrage is opposed by its enemies might assuage these fears. If, as we are told, women will not take the pains to vote except upon the strongest inducements, who has so good an opportunity as the husband to bring those inducements to bear? and, if so, what is the separation? Or if, as we are told, women will merely reflect their husbands' political opinions, why should they dispute about them? The mere suggestion of a difference deep enough to quarrel for, implies a real difference of convictions or interests, and indicates that there ought to be an independent representation of each; unless we fall back, once for all, on the common-law tradition that man and wife are one, and that one is the husband. Either the antagonisms which occur in politics are comparatively superficial, in which case they would do no harm; or else they touch matters of real interest and principle, in which case every human being has a right to independent expression, even at a good deal of risk. In either case, the objection falls to the ground.

We have fortunately a means of testing, with some fairness of estimate, the probable amount of this peril. It is generally admitted,—and certainly no German-American will deny,—that the most fruitful sources of hostility and war in all times have been religious, not political. All merely political antagonism, certainly all which is possible in a republic, fades into insignificance before this more powerful dividing influence. Yet we leave all this great explosive force in unimpeded operation,—at any moment it may be set in action, in any one of those "pretty family scenes" which "Puck" depicts,—while we are solemnly warned against admitting the comparatively mild peril of a political difference! It is like cautioning a manufacturer of dynamite against the danger of meddling with mere edge-tools. Even with all the intensity of feeling on religious matters, few families are seriously divided by them; and the influence of political differences would be still more insignificant.

The simple fact is, that there is no better basis for union than mutual respect for each other's opinions; and this can never be obtained without an intelligent independence. "I would rather have a thorn in my side than an echo," said Emerson of friendship; and the same is true of married life. It is the echoes, the nonentities, of whom men grow tired; it is the women with some flavor of individuality who keep the hearts of their husbands. This is only applying in a higher sense what Shakspeare's Cleopatra saw. When her handmaidens are questioning how to hold a lover, and one says,—

"Give way to him in all: cross him in nothing,"—

Cleopatra, from the depth of an unequalled experience, retorts,—

"Thou speakest like a fool: the way to lose him!"

And what "the serpent of old Nile" said, the wives of the future, who are to be wise as serpents and harmless as doves, may well ponder. It takes two things different to make a union; and part of that difference may as well lie in matters political as anywhere else.

XXXI.
WOMEN AS ECONOMISTS.

An able lawyer of Boston, arguing the other day before a legislative committee in favor of giving to the city council a check upon the expenditures of the school committee, gave as one reason that this body would probably include more women henceforward, and that women were ordinarily more lavish than men in their use of money. The truth of this assumption was questioned at the time: and, the more I think of it, the more contrary it is to my whole experience. I should say that women, from the very habit of their lives, are led to be more particular about details, and more careful as to small economies. The very fact that they handle less money tends to this. When they are told to spend money, as they often are by loving or ambitious husbands, they no doubt do it freely: they have naturally more taste than men, and quite as much love of luxury. In some instances in this country they spend money recklessly and wickedly, like the heroines of French novels; but as, even in brilliant Paris, the women of the middle classes are notoriously better managers than the men, so we often see, in our scheming America, the same relative superiority. Often have I heard young men say, "I never knew how to economize until after my marriage;" and who has not seen multitudes of instances where women accustomed to luxury have accepted poverty without a murmur for the sake of those whom they loved?

I remember a young girl, accustomed to the gayest society of New York, who engaged herself to a young naval officer, against the advice of the friends of both. One of her near relatives said to me, "Of all the young girls I have ever known, she is the least fitted for a poor man's wife." Yet from the very moment of her marriage she brought their joint expenses within his scanty pay, and even saved a little money from it. Everybody knows such instances. We hear men denounce the extravagance of women, while those very men spend on wine and cigars, on clubs and horses, twice what their wives spend on their toilet. If the wives are economical, the husbands perhaps urge them on to greater lavishness. "Why do you not dress like Mrs. So-and-so?"—"I can't afford it."—"But *I* can afford it;" and then, when the bills come in, the talk of extravagance recommences. At one time in Newport that lady among the summer visitors who was reported to be

Worth's best customer was also well known to be quite indifferent to society, and to go into it mainly to please her husband, whose social ambition was notorious.

It has often happened to me to serve in organizations where both sexes were represented, and where expenditures were to be made for business or pleasure. In these I have found, as a rule, that the women were more careful, or perhaps I should say more timid, than the men, less willing to risk any thing: the bolder financial experiments came from the men, as one might expect. In talking the other day with the secretary of an important educational enterprise, conducted by women, I was surprised to find that it was cramped for money, though large subscriptions were said to have been made to it. On inquiry it appeared that these ladies, having pledged themselves for four years, had divided the amount received into four parts, and were resolutely limiting themselves, for the first year, to one quarter part of what had been subscribed. No board of men would have done so. Any board of men would have allowed far more than a quarter of the sum for the first year's expenditures, justly reasoning that if the enterprise began well it would command public confidence, and bring in additional subscriptions as time went on. I would appeal to any one whose experience has been in joint associations of men and women, whether this is not a fair statement of the difference between their ways of working. It does not prove that women are more honest than men, but that their education or their nature makes them more cautious in expenditure.

The habits of society make the dress of a fashionable woman far more expensive than that of a man of fashion. Formerly it was not so; and, so long as it was not so, the extravagance of men in this respect quite equalled that of women. It now takes other forms, but the habit is the same. There is not a club-house in Boston furnished with such absence of luxury as the Women's Club rooms on Park Street: the contrast was at first so great as to seem almost absurd. The waiters at any fashionable restaurant will tell you that what is a cheap dinner for a man would be a dear dinner for a woman. Yet after all, the test is not in any particular class of expenditures, but in the business-like habit. Men are of course more business-like in large combinations, for they are more used to them; but for the small details of daily economy women are more watchful. The cases where women ruin their husbands by extravagance are exceptional. As a rule, the men are the bread-winners; but the careful saving and managing and contriving come from the women.

XXXII.
GREATER INCLUDES LESS.

I was once at a little musical party in New York, where several accomplished amateur singers were present, and with them the eminent professional, Miss Adelaide Phillips. The amateurs were first called on. Each chose some difficult operatic passage, and sang her best. When it came to the great opera-singer's turn, instead of exhibiting her ability to eclipse those rivals on her own ground, she simply seated herself at the piano, and sang "Kathleen Mavourneen" with such thrilling sweetness, that the young Irish girl who was setting the supper-table in the next room forgot all her plates and teaspoons, threw herself into a chair, put her apron over her face, and sobbed as if her heart would break. All the training of Adelaide Phillips—her magnificent voice, her stage experience, her skill in effects, her power of expression—went into the performance of that simple song. The greater included the less. And thus all the intellectual and practical training that any woman can have, all her public action and her active career, will make her, if she be a true woman, more admirable as a wife, a mother, and a friend. The greater includes the less for her also.

Of course this is a statement of general facts and tendencies. There must be among women, as among men, an endless variety of individual temperaments. There will always be plenty whose career will illustrate the infirmities of genius, and whom no training can convince that two and two make four. But the general fact is sure. As no sensible man would seriously prefer for a wife a Hindoo or Tahitian woman rather than one bred in England or America, so every further advantage of education or opportunity will only improve, not impair, the true womanly type.

Lucy Stone once said, "Woman's nature was stamped and sealed by the Almighty, and there is no danger of her unsexing herself while his eye watches her." Margaret Fuller said, "One hour of love will teach a woman more of her true relations than all your philosophizing." These were the testimony of women who had studied Greek, and were only the more womanly for the study. They are worth the opinions of a million half-developed beings like the Duchess de Fontanges, who was described as being "as beautiful as an angel and as silly as a goose." The greater includes the less. Your view from the mountain-side may be very pretty, but she who has taken one step higher commands your view and her own also. It was no dreamy recluse, but the accomplished and experienced Stendhal, who wrote, "The joys of the gay world do not count for much with happy women."[7]

7. De l'Amour, par de Stendhal (Henri Beyle): "Les plaisirs du grand monde n'en sont pas pour les femmes heureuses," p. 189.

If a highly educated man is incapable and unpractical, we do not say that he is educated too well, but not well enough. He ought to know what he knows, and other things also. Never yet did I see a woman too well educated to be a wife and a mother; but I know multitudes who deplore, or have reason to deplore, every day of their lives, the untrained and unfurnished minds that are so ill-prepared for these sacred duties. Every step towards equalizing the opportunities of men and women meets with resistance, of course; but every step, as it is accomplished, leaves men still men, and women still women. And as we who heard Adelaide Phillips felt that she had never had a better tribute to her musical genius than that young Irish girl's tears; so the true woman will feel that all her college training for instance, if she has it, may have been well invested, even for the sake of the baby on her knee. And it is to be remembered, after all, that each human being lives to unfold his or her own powers, and do his or her own duties first, and that neither woman nor man has the right to accept a merely secondary and subordinate life. A noble woman must be a noble human being; and the most sacred special duties, as of wife or mother, are all included in this, as the greater includes the less.

XXXIII.
A CO-PARTNERSHIP.

Marriage, considered merely in its financial and business relations, may be regarded as a permanent co-partnership.

Now, in an ordinary co-partnership, there is very often a complete division of labor among the partners. If they manufacture locomotive-engines, for instance, one partner perhaps superintends the works, another attends to mechanical inventions and improvements, another travels for orders, another conducts the correspondence, another receives and pays out the money. The latter is not necessarily the head of the firm. Perhaps his place could be more easily filled than some of the other posts. Nevertheless, more money passes through his hands than through those of all the others put together. Now, should he, at the year's end, call together the inventor and the superintendent and the traveller and the correspondent, and say to them, "I have earned all this money this year, but I will generously give you some of it,"—he would be considered simply impertinent, and would hardly have a chance to repeat the offence, the year after.

Yet precisely what would be called folly in this business partnership is constantly done by men in the co-partnership of marriage, and is there called "common-sense" and "social science" and "political economy."

For instance, a farmer works himself half to death in the hay-field, and his wife meanwhile is working herself wholly to death in the dairy. The neighbors come in to sympathize after her demise; and, during the few months' interval before his second marriage, they say approvingly, "He was always a generous man to his folks! He was a good provider!" But where was the room for generosity, any more than the member of any other firm is to be called generous, when he keeps the books, receipts the bills, and divides the money?

In case of the farming business, the share of the wife is so direct and unmistakable that it can hardly be evaded. If any thing is earned by the farm, she does her distinct and important share of the earning. But it is not necessary that she should do even that, to make her, by all the rules of justice, an equal partner, entitled to her full share of the financial proceeds.

Let us suppose an ordinary case. Two young people are married, and begin life together. Let us suppose them equally poor, equally capable, equally conscientious, equally healthy. They have children. Those children must be supported by the earning of money abroad, by attendance and care at home. If it requires patience and labor to do the outside work, no less is required inside. The duties of the household are as hard as the duties of the shop or office. If the wife took her husband's work for a day, she would probably be glad to return to her own. So would the husband if he undertook hers. Their duties are ordinarily as distinct and as equal as those of two partners in any other co-partnership. It so happens, that the out-door partner has the handling of the money; but does that give him a right to claim it as his exclusive earnings? No more than in any other business operation.

He earned the money for the children and the household. She disbursed it for the children and the household. The very laws of nature, by giving her the children to bear and rear, absolve her from the duty of their support, so long as he is alive who was left free by nature for that purpose. Her task on the average is as hard as his: nay, a portion of it is so especially hard that it is distinguished from all others by the name "labor." If it does not earn money, it is because it is not to be measured in money, while it exists—nor to be replaced by money, if lost. If a business man loses his partner, he can obtain another: and a man, no doubt, may take a second wife; but he cannot procure for his children a second mother. Indeed, it is a palpable insult to the whole relation of husband and wife when one compares it, even in a financial light, to that of business partners. It is only because a constant effort is made to degrade the practical position of woman below even this standard of comparison, that it becomes her duty to claim for herself at least as much as this.

There was a tradition in a town where I once lived, that a certain Quaker, who had married a fortune, was once heard to repel his wife, who had asked him for money in a public place, with the response, "Rachel, where is that ninepence I gave thee yesterday?" When I read in Scribner's Monthly an article deriding the right to representation of the Massachusetts women who pay two millions of tax on one hundred and thirty-two million dollars of property,—asserting that they produced nothing of it; that it was only "men who produced this wealth, and bestowed it upon these women;" that it was "all drawn from land and sea by the hands of men whose largess testifies alike of their love and their munificence,"—I must say that I am reminded of Rachel's ninepence.

XXXIV.
"ONE RESPONSIBLE HEAD."

When we look through any business directory, there seem to be almost as many co-partnerships as single dealers; and three-quarters of these co-partnerships appear to consist of precisely two persons, no more, no less. These partners are, in the eye of the law, equal. It is not found necessary under the law, to make a general provision that in each case one partner should be supreme and the other subordinate. In many cases, by the terms of the co-partnership there are limitations on one side and special privileges on the other,—marriage settlements, as it were; but the general law of co-partnership is based on the presumption of equality. It would be considered infinitely absurd to require, that, as the general rule, one party or the other should be in a state of *coverture*, during which the very being and existence of the one should be suspended, or entirely merged and incorporated into that of the other.

And yet this requirement, which would be an admitted absurdity in the case of two business partners, is precisely that which the English common law still lays down in case of husband and wife. The words which I employed to describe it, in the preceding sentence, are the very phrases in which Blackstone describes the legal position of women. And though the English common law has been, in this respect, greatly modified and superseded by statute law; yet, when it comes to an argument on woman suffrage, it is constantly this same tradition to which men and even women habitually appeal,—the necessity of a single head to the domestic partnership, and the necessity that the husband should be that head. This is especially true of English men and women; but it is true of Americans as well. Nobody has stated it more tersely than Fitzjames Stephen, in his "Liberty, Equality, and Fraternity" (p. 216), when arguing against Mr. Mill's view of the equality of the sexes.

"Marriage is a contract, one of the principal objects in which is the government of a family.

"This government must be vested, either by law or by contract, in the hands of one of the two married persons."

[Then follow some collateral points, not bearing on the present question.]

"Therefore if marriage is to be permanent, the government of the family must be put by law and by morals into the hands of the husband, for no one proposes to give it to the wife."

This argument he calls "as clear as that of a proposition in Euclid." He thinks that the business of life can be carried on by no other method. How is it, then, that when we come to what is called technically and especially the "business" of every day, this whole finespun theory is disregarded, and men come together in partnership on the basis of equality?

Nobody is farther than I from regarding marriage as a mere business partnership. But it is to be observed that the points wherein it differs from a merely mercantile connection are points that should make equality more easy, not more difficult. The tie between two ordinary business partners is merely one of interest: it is based on no sentiments, sealed by no solemn pledge, enriched by no home associations, cemented by no new generation of young life. If a relation like this is found to work well on terms of equality,—so well that a large part of the business of the world is done by it,—is it not absurd to suppose that the same equal relation cannot exist in the married partnership of husband and wife? And if law, custom, society, all recognize this fact of equality in the one case, why, in the name of common-sense, should they not equally recognize it in the other?

And, again, it must be far easier to assign a sphere to each partner in marriage than in business; and therefore the double headship of a family will involve less need of collision. In nine cases out of ten, the external support of the family can devolve upon the husband, unquestioned by the wife; and its internal economy upon the wife, unquestioned by the husband. No voluntary distribution of powers and duties between business partners can work so naturally, on the whole, as this simple and easy demarcation, with which the claim of suffrage makes no necessary interference. It may require angry discussion to decide which of two business partners shall buy, and which shall sell; which shall keep the books, and which do the active work, and so on; but all this is usually settled in married life by the natural order of things. Even in regard to the management of children, where collision is likely to come, if anywhere, it can commonly be settled by that happy formula of Jean Paul's, that the mother usually supplies the commas and the semicolons in the child's book of life, and the father the colons and periods. And as to matters in general, the simple and practical rule, that each question that arises should be decided by that partner who has personally most at stake in it, will, in ninety-nine times out of a hundred, carry the domestic partnership through without shipwreck. Those who cannot meet the hundredth case by mutual forbearance are in a condition of shipwreck already.

XXXV.
ASKING FOR MONEY.

One of the very best wives and mothers I have ever known once said to me, that, whenever her daughters should be married, she should stipulate in their behalf with their husbands for a regular sum of money to be paid them, at certain intervals, for their personal expenditures. Whether this sum was to be larger or smaller, was a matter of secondary importance,—that must depend on the income, and the style of living; but the essential thing was, that it should come to the wife regularly, so that she should no more have to make a special request for it than her husband would have to ask her for a dinner. This lady's own husband was, as I happened to know, of a most generous disposition, was devotedly attached to her, and denied her nothing. She herself was a most accurate and careful manager. There was every thing in the household to make the financial arrangements flow smoothly. Yet she said to me, "I suppose no man can possibly understand how a sensitive woman shrinks from *asking* for money. If I can prevent it, my daughters shall never have to ask for it. If they do their duty as wives and mothers they have a right to their share of the joint income, within reasonable limits; for certainly no money could buy the services they render. Moreover, they have a right to a share in determining what those reasonable limits are."

Now, it so happened that I had myself gone through an experience which enabled me perfectly to comprehend this feeling. In early life I was for a time in the employ of one of my relatives, who paid me a fair salary but at no definite periods: I was at liberty to ask him for money up to a certain amount whenever I needed it. This seemed to me, in advance, a most agreeable arrangement; but I found it quite otherwise. It proved to be very disagreeable to ask for money: it made every dollar seem a special favor; it brought up all kinds of misgivings, as to whether he could spare it without inconvenience, whether he really thought my services worth it, and so on. My employer was a thoroughly upright and noble man, and I was much attached to him. I do not know that he ever refused or demurred when I asked for money. The annoyance was simply in the process of asking; and this became so great, that I often underwent serious inconvenience rather than ask. Finally, at the year's end, I surprised my relative very much by saying that I would accept, if necessary, a lower salary, on condition that it should be paid on regular days, and as a matter of business. The wish was at once granted, without the reduction; and he probably never knew what a relief it was to me.

Now, if a young man is liable to feel this pride and reluctance toward an employer, even if a kinsman, it is easy to understand how many women may feel the same, even in regard to a husband. And I fancy that those who feel it most are often the most conscientious and high-minded women. It is unreasonable to say of such persons, "Too sensitive! Too fastidious!" For it is just this quality of finer sensitiveness which men affect to prize in a woman, and wish to protect at all hazards. The very fact that a husband is generous; the very fact that his income is limited,—these may bring in conscience and gratitude to increase the restraining influence of pride, and make the wife less willing to ask money of such a husband than if he were a rich man or a mean one. The only dignified position in which a man can place his wife is to treat her at least as well as he would treat a housekeeper, and give her the comfort of a perfectly clear and definite arrangement as to money matters. She will not then be under the necessity of nerving herself to solicit from him as a favor what she really needs and has a right to spend. Nor will she be torturing herself, on the other side, with the secret fear lest she has asked too much and more than they can really spare. She will, in short, be in the position of a woman and a wife, not of a child or a toy.

I have carefully avoided using the word "allowance" in what has been said, because that word seems to imply the untrue and mean assumption that the money is all the husband's to give or withhold as he will. Yet I have heard this sort of phrase from men who were living on a wife's property or a wife's earnings; from men who nominally kept boarding-houses, working a little, while their wives worked hard,—or from farmers, who worked hard, and made their wives work harder. Even in cases where the wife has no direct part in the money-making, the indirect part she performs, if she takes faithful charge of her household, is so essential, so beyond all compensation in money, that it is an utter shame and impertinence in the husband when he speaks of "giving" money to his wife as if it were an act of favor. It is no more an act of favor than when the business manager of a firm pays out money to the unseen partner who directs the indoor business or runs the machinery. Be the joint income more or less, the wife has a claim to her honorable share, and that as a matter of right, without the daily ignominy of sending in a petition for it.

XXXVI.
WOMANHOOD AND MOTHERHOOD.

I always groan in spirit when any advocate of woman suffrage, carried away by zeal, says any thing disrespectful about the nursery. It is contrary to the general tone of feeling among us, I am sure, to speak of this priceless institution as a trivial or degrading sphere, unworthy the emancipated woman. It is rarely that anybody speaks in this way; but a single such utterance hurts us more than any arguments of the enemy. For every thoughtful person sees that the cares of motherhood, though not the whole duty of woman, are an essential part of that duty, wherever they occur; and that no theory of womanly life is good for any thing which undertakes to leave out the cradle. Even her school-education is based on this fact, were it only on Stendhal's theory that the sons of a woman who reads Gibbon and Schiller will be more likely to show talent than those of one who only tells her beads and reads Mme. de Genlis. And so clearly is this understood among us, that, when we ask for suffrage for woman, it is almost always claimed that she needs it for the sake of her children. To secure her in her right to them; to give her a voice in their education; to give her a vote in the government beneath which they are to live,—these points are seldom omitted in our statement of her claims. Any thing else would be an error.

But there is an error at the other extreme, which is still greater. A woman should no more merge herself in her child than in her husband. Yet we often hear that she should do just this. What is all the public sphere of woman, it is said,—what good can she do by all her speaking, and writing, and action, —compared with that she does by properly training the soul of one child? It is not easy to see the logic of this claim.

For of what service is that child to be in the universe, except that he, too, may write and speak and act for that which is good and true? And if the mother foregoes all this that the child, in growing up, may simply do what the mother has left undone, the world gains nothing. In sacrificing her own work to her child's, moreover, she exchanges a present good for a prospective and merely possible one. If she does this through overwhelming love, we can hardly blame her; but she cannot justify it before reason and truth. Her child may die, and the service to mankind be done by neither. Her child may grow up with talents unlike hers, or with none at all; as the son of

Howard was selfish, the son of Chesterfield a boor, and the son of Wordsworth in the last degree prosaic.

Or the special occasion when she might have done great good may have passed before her boy or girl grows up to do it. If Mrs. Child had refused to write "An Appeal for that Class of Americans called Africans," or Mrs. Stowe had laid aside "Uncle Tom's Cabin," or Florence Nightingale had declined to go to the Crimea, on the ground that a woman's true work was through the nursery, and they must all wait for that, the consequence would be that these things would have remained undone. The brave acts of the world must be done when occasion offers, by the first brave soul who feels moved to do them, man or woman. If all the children in all the nurseries are thereby helped to do other brave deeds when their turn comes, so much the better. But when a great opportunity offers for direct aid to the world, we have no right to transfer that work to other hands—not even to the hands of our own children. We must do the work, and train the children besides.

I am willing to admit, therefore, that the work of education, in any form, is as great as any other work; but I fail to see why it should be greater. Usefulness is usefulness: there is no reason why it should be postponed from generation to generation, or why it is better to rear a serviceable human being than to be one in person. Carry the theory consistently out: each mother must simply rear her daughter that she in turn may rear somebody else; from each generation the work will devolve upon a succeeding generation, so that it will be only the last woman who will personally do any service, except that of motherhood; and when her time comes it will be too late for any service at all.

If it be said, "But some of these children will be men, who are necessarily of more use than women," I deny the necessity. If it be said, "The children may be many, and the mother, who is but one, may well be sacrificed," it might be replied, that as one great act may be worth many smaller ones, so all the numerous children and grandchildren of a woman like Lucretia Mott may not collectively equal the usefulness of herself alone. If she, like many women, had held it her duty to renounce all other duties and interests from the time her motherhood began, I think that the world, and even her children, would have lost more than ever could have been gained by her more complete absorption in the nursery.

The true theory seems a very simple one. The very fact that during one-half the years of a woman's average life she is made incapable of child-bearing, shows that there are, even for the most prolific and devoted mothers, duties other than the maternal. Even during the most absorbing years of motherhood, the wisest women still try to keep up their interest in society, in literature, in the world's affairs—were it only for their children's sake. Multitudes of women will never be mothers; and those more fortunate may find even the usefulness of their motherhood surpassed by what they do in other ways. If maternal duties interfere in some degree with all other functions, the same is true, though in a far less degree, of those of a father. But there are those who combine both spheres. The German poet Wieland claimed to be the parent of fourteen children and forty books; and who knows by which parentage he served the world the best?

XXXVII.
A GERMAN POINT OF VIEW.

Many Americans will remember the favorable impression made by Professor Christlieb of Germany, when he attended the meeting of the Evangelical Alliance in New York some four or five years ago. His writings, like his presence, show a most liberal spirit; and perhaps no man has ever presented the more advanced evangelical theology of Germany in so attractive a light. Yet I heard a story of him the other day, which either showed him in an aspect quite undesirable, or else gave a disagreeable view of the social position of women in Germany.

The story was to the effect, that a young American student recently called on Professor Christlieb with a letter of introduction. The professor received him cordially, and soon entered into conversation about the United States. He praised the natural features of the country, and the enterprising spirit of our citizens, but expressed much solicitude about the future of the nation. On being asked his reasons, he frankly expressed his opinion that "the Spirit of Christ" was not here. Being still further pressed to illustrate his meaning, he gave, as instances of this deficiency, not the Crédit Mobilier or the Tweed scandal, but such alarming facts as the following. He seriously declared, that, on more than one occasion, he had heard an American married woman say to her husband, "Dear, will you bring me my shawl?" and the husband had brought it. He further had seen a husband return home at evening, and enter the parlor where his wife was sitting,—perhaps in the very best chair in the room,—and the wife not only did not go and get his dressing-gown and slippers, but she even remained seated, and left him to find a chair as he could. These things, as Professor Christlieb pointed out, suggested a serious deficiency of the Spirit of Christ in the community.

With our American habits and interpretations, it is hard to see this matter just as the professor sees it. One would suppose, that, if there is any meaning in the command, "Bear ye one another's burdens, and so fulfil the law of Christ," a little of such fulfilling might sometimes be good for the husband, as for the wife. And though it would undoubtedly be more pleasing to see every wife so eager to receive her husband that she would naturally spring from her chair and run to kiss him in the doorway, yet, where such devotion was wanting, it would be but fair to inquire which of the two had had the more fatiguing day's work, and to whom the easy-chair justly belonged. The truth is, I suppose, that the good professor's remark indicated simply a "survival" in his mind, or in his social circle, of a barbarous tradition, under which the wife of a Mexican herdsman cannot eat at the table with her "lord and master," and the wife of a German professor must vacate the best arm-chair at his approach.

If so, it is not to be regretted that we in this country have outgrown a relation so unequal. Nor am I at all afraid that the great Teacher, who, pointing to the multitude for whom he was soon to die, said of them, "This is my brother and my sister and my mother," would have objected to any mutual and equal service between man and woman. If we assume that two human beings have immortal souls, there can be no want of dignity to either in serving the other. The greater equality of woman in America seems to be, on this reasoning, a proof of the presence, not the absence, of the spirit of Christ; nor does Dr. Christlieb seem to me quite worthy of the beautiful name he bears, if he feels otherwise.

But, if it is really true that a German professor has to cross the Atlantic to witness a phenomenon so very simple as that of a lover-like husband bringing a shawl for his wife, I should say, Let the immigration from Germany be encouraged as much as possible, in order that even the most learned immigrants may discover something new.

XXXVIII.
CHILDLESS WOMEN.

It has not always been regarded as a thing creditable to woman, that she was the mother of the human race. On the contrary, the fact was often mentioned, in the Middle Ages, as a distinct proof of inferiority. The question was discussed in the mediæval Council of Mâcon, and the position taken that woman was no more entitled to rank as human, because she brought forth men, than the garden-earth could take rank with the fruit and flowers it bore. The same view was revived by a Latin writer of 1595, on the thesis *"Mulieres non homines esse,"* a French translation of which essay was printed under the title of *"Paradoxe sur les femmes,"* in 1766. Napoleon Bonaparte used the same image, carrying it almost as far:—

"Woman is given to man that she may bear children. Woman is our property; we are not hers: because she produces children for us; we do not yield any to her: she is therefore our possession, as the fruit-tree is that of the gardener."

Even the fact of parentage, therefore, has been adroitly converted into a ground of inferiority for women; and this is ostensibly the reason why lineage has been reckoned, almost everywhere, through the male line only, ignoring the female; just as, in tracing the seed of some rare fruit, the gardener takes no genealogical account of the garden where it grew. The view is now seldom expressed in full force: the remnant of it is to be found in the lingering impression, that, at any rate, a woman who is not a mother is of no account; as worthless as a fruitless garden or a barren fruit-tree. Created only for a certain object, she is of course valueless unless that object be fulfilled.

But the race must have fathers as well as mothers; and, if we look for evidence of public service in great men, it certainly does not always lie in leaving children to the republic. On the contrary, the rule has rather seemed to be, that the most eminent men have left their bequest of service in any form rather than in that of a great family. Recent inquiries into the matter have brought out some remarkable facts in this regard.

As a rule, there exist no living descendants in the male line from the great authors, artists, statesmen, soldiers, of England. It is stated that there is not one such descendant of Chaucer, Shakespeare, Spenser, Butler, Dryden, Pope, Cowper, Goldsmith, Scott, Byron, or Moore; not one of Drake, Cromwell, Monk, Marlborough, Peterborough, or Nelson; not one of Strafford, Ormond, or Clarendon; not one of Addison, Swift, or Johnson; not one of Walpole, Bolingbroke, Chatham, Pitt, Fox, Burke, Grattan, or Canning; not one of Bacon, Locke, Newton, or Davy; not one of Hume, Gibbon, or Macaulay; not one of Hogarth or Reynolds; not one of Garrick, John Kemble, or Edmund Kean. It would be easy to make a similar American list, beginning with Washington, of whom it was said that "Providence made him childless that his country might call him Father."

Now, however we may regret that these great men have left little or no posterity, it does not occur to any one as affording any serious drawback upon their service to their nation. Certainly it does not occur to us that they would have been more useful had they left children to the world, but rendered it no other service. Lord Bacon says that "he that hath wife and children hath given hostages to fortune; for they are impediments to great enterprises, either of virtue or mischief. Certainly the best works, and of greatest merit to the public, have proceeded from unmarried or childless men; which, both in affection and means, have married and endowed the public." And this is the view generally accepted,—that the public is in such cases rather the gainer than the loser, and has no right to complain.

Since, therefore, every child must have a father and a mother both, and neither will alone suffice, why should we thus heap gratitude on men who from preference or from necessity have remained childless, and yet habitually treat women as if they could render no service to their country except by giving it children? If it be folly and shame, as I think, to belittle and decry the dignity and worth of motherhood, as some are said to do, it is no less folly, and shame quite as great, to deny the grand and patriotic service of many women who have died and left no children among their mourners. Plato puts into the mouth of a woman,—the eloquent Diotima, in the "Banquet,"—that, after all, we are more grateful to Homer and Hesiod for the children of their brain than if they had left human offspring.

XXXIX.
THE PREVENTION OF CRUELTY TO MOTHERS.

From the Society for the Prevention of Cruelty to Animals we have now advanced to a similar society for the benefit of children. When shall we have a movement for the prevention of cruelty to mothers?

A Rhode Island lady, who had never taken any interest in the woman suffrage movement, came to me in great indignation the other day, asking if it was true that under Rhode Island laws a husband might, by his last will, bequeath his child away from its mother, so that she might, if the guardian chose, never see it again. I said that it was undoubtedly true, and that such were still the laws in many States of the Union.

"But," she said, "it is an outrage. The husband may have been one of the weakest or worst men in the world; he may have persecuted his wife and children; he may have made the will in a moment of anger, and have neglected to alter it. At any rate, he is dead, and the mother is living. The guardian whom he appoints may turn out a very malicious man, and may take pleasure in torturing the mother; or he may bring up the children in a way their mother thinks ruinous for them. Why do not all the mothers cry out against such a law?"

"I wish they would," I said. "I have been trying a good many years to make them even understand what the law is; but they do not. People who do not vote pay no attention to the laws, until they suffer from them."

She went away protesting that she, at least, would not hold her tongue on the subject, and I hope she will not. The actual text of the law is as follows:

"Every person authorized by law to make a will, except married women, shall have a right to appoint by his will a guardian or guardians for his children during their minority."[8]

[8]. Gen. Statutes R. I., chap. 154, sect. 1.

There is not associated with this, in the statute, the slightest clause in favor of the mother; nor any thing which could limit the power of the guardian by requiring deference to her wishes, although he could, in case of gross neglect or abuse, be removed by the court, and another guardian appointed. There is not a line of positive law to protect the mother. Now, in a case of absolute wrong, a single sentence of law is worth all the chivalrous courtesy this side of the Middle Ages.

It is idle to say that such laws are not executed. They are executed. I have had letters, too agonizing to print, expressing the sufferings of mothers under laws like these. There lies before me a letter,—not from Rhode Island,—written by a widowed mother who suffers daily tortures, even while in possession of her child, at the knowledge that it is not legally hers, but held only by the temporary permission of the guardian appointed under her husband's will. "I beg you," she says, "to take this will to the hill-top, and urge law-makers in our next Legislature to free the State record from the shameful story that no mother can control her child unless it is born out of wedlock."

"From the moment," she says, "when the will was read to me, I have made no effort to set it aside. I wait till God reveals his plans, so far as my own condition is concerned. But out of my keen comprehension of this great wrong, notwithstanding my submission for myself, my whole soul is stirred,—for my child, who is a little woman; for all women, that the laws may be changed which subject a true woman, a devoted wife, a faithful mother, to such mental agonies as I have endured, and shall endure till I die."

In a later letter she says, "I now have his [the guardian's] solemn promise that he will not remove her from my control. To some extent my sufferings are allayed; and yet never, till she arrives at the age of twenty-one, shall I fully trust." I wish that mothers who dwell in sheltered and happy homes would try to bring to their minds the condition of a mother whose possession of her only child rests upon the "promise" of a comparative stranger. We should get beyond the meaningless cry, "I have all the rights I want," if mothers could only remember that among these rights, in most States of the Union, the right of a widowed mother to her child is not included.

By strenuous effort, the law on this point has in Massachusetts been gradually amended, till it now stands thus: The father is authorized to appoint a guardian by will; but the powers of this guardian do not entitle him to take the child from the mother.

"The guardian of a minor ... shall have the custody and tuition of his ward; and the care and management of all his estate, except that the father of the minor, if living, and in case of his death the mother, they being respectively competent to transact their own business, shall be entitled to the custody of the person of the minor and the care of his education."[9]

9. Public Statutes, chap. 139, sect. 4.

Down to 1870 the cruel words "while she remains unmarried" followed the word "mother" in the above law. Until that time, the mother if remarried had no claim to the custody of her child, in case the guardian wished otherwise; and a very painful scene once took place in a Boston court-room, where children were forced away from their mother by the officers, under this statute; in spite of her tears and theirs; and this when no sort of personal charge had been made against her. This could not now happen in Massachusetts, but it might still happen in some other States. It is true that men are almost always better than their laws; but, while a bad law remains on the statute-book, it gives to any unscrupulous man the power to be as bad as the law.

SOCIETY.

"Place the sexes in right relations of mutual respect, and a severe morality gives that essential charm to woman which educates all that is delicate, poetic, and self-sacrificing, breeds courtesy and learning, conversation and wit, in her rough mate; so that I have thought a sufficient measure of civilization is the influence of good women."—EMERSON: *Society and Solitude*, p. 21.

XL.
FOAM AND CURRENT.

Sometimes, on the beach at Newport, I look at the gayly dressed ladies in their phaëtons, and then at the foam which trembles on the breaking wave, or lies palpitating in creamy masses on the beach. It is as pretty as they, as light, as fresh, as delicate, as changing; and no doubt the graceful foam, if it thinks at all, fancies that it is the chief consummate product of the ocean, and that the main end of the vast currents of the mighty deep is to yield a few glittering bubbles like those. At least, this seems to me what many of the fair ladies think.

Here is a nation in which the most momentous social and political experiment ever tried by man is being worked out, day by day. There is something oceanlike in the way in which the great currents of life, race, religion, temperament, are here chafing with each other, safe from the storms through which all monarchical countries may yet have to pass. As these great currents heave, there are tossed up in every watering-place and every city in America, as on an ocean-beach, certain pretty bubbles of foam; and each spot, we may suppose, counts its own bubbles brighter than those of its neighbors, and christens them "society."

It is an unceasing wonder to a thoughtful person, at any such resort, to see the unconscious way in which fashionable society accepts the foam, and ignores the currents. You hear people talk of "a position in society," "the influential circles in society," as if the position they mean were not liable to be shifted in a day; as if the essential influences in America were not mainly to be sought outside the world of fashion. In other countries it is very different. The circle of social caste, whose centre you touch in London, radiates to the shores of the island; the upper class controls, not merely fashion, but government; it rules in country as well as city; genius and wealth are but its tributaries. Wherever it is not so, it is because England is so far Americanized. But in America the social prestige of the cities is nothing in the country; it is a matter of the pavement, of a three-mile radius.

Go to the farthest borders of England: there are still the "county families," and you meet servants in livery. On the other hand, in a little village in Northern New Hampshire, my friend was visited in the evening by the landlady, who said that several of their "most fashionable ladies" had happened in, and she would like to exhibit to them her guest's bonnet. Then the different cities ignore each other: the rulers of select circles in New York find themselves nobodies in Washington, while a Washington social passport counts for as little in New York. Boston and Philadelphia affect to ignore both; and St. Louis and San Francisco have their own standards. The utmost social prestige in America is local, provincial, a matter of the square inch: it is as if the foam of each particular beach along the seacoast were to call itself "society."

There is something pathetic, therefore, in the unwearied pains taken by ambitious women to establish a place in some little, local, transitory domain, to "bring out" their daughters for exhibition on a given evening, to form a circle for them, to marry them well. A dozen years hence the millionnaires whose notice they seek may be paupers, or these ladies may be dwelling in some other city, where the visiting cards will bear wholly different names. How idle to attempt to transport into American life the social traditions and delusions which require monarchy and primogeniture, and a standing army, to keep them up—and which cannot hold their own in England, even with the aid of these!

Every woman, like every man, has a natural desire for influence; and if this instinct yearns, as it often should yearn, to take in more than her own family, she must seek it somewhere outside. I know women who bring to bear on the building-up of a frivolous social circle—frivolous, because it is not really brilliant, but only showy; not really gay, but only bored—talent and energy enough to influence the mind and thought of the nation, if only employed in some effective way. Who are the women of real influence in America? They are the school-teachers, through whose hands each successive American generation has to pass; they are those wives of public men who share their husbands' labor, and help mould their work; they are those women, who, through their personal eloquence or through the press, are distinctly influencing the American people in its growth. The influence of such women is felt for good or for evil in every page they print, every newspaper-column they fill: the individual women may be unworthy their posts, but it is they who have got hold of the lever, and gone the right way to work. As American society is constituted, the largest "social success" that can be attained here is trivial and local; and you have to "make believe very hard," like that other imaginary Marchioness, to find in it any career worth mentioning. That is the foam, but these other women are dealing with the main currents.

XLI.
"IN SOCIETY."

One sometimes hears from some lady the remark that very few people "in society" believe in any movement to enlarge the rights or duties of women. In a community of more marked social gradations than our own, this assertion, if true, might be very important; and even here it is worth considering, because it leads the way to a little social philosophy. Let us, for the sake of argument, begin by accepting the assumption that there is an inner circle, at least in our large cities, which claims to be "society," *par excellence*. What relation has this favored circle, if favored it be, to any movement relating to women?

It has, to begin with, the same relation that "society" has to every movement of reform. The proportion of smiles and frowns offered from this quarter to the woman-suffrage movement, for instance, is about that offered to the anti-slavery agitation: I see no great difference. In Boston, for example, the names contributed by "society" to the woman-suffrage festivals are about as numerous as those formerly contributed to the anti-slavery bazaars; no more, no less. Indeed, they are very often the same names; and it has been curious to see, for nearly fifty years, how radical tendencies have predominated in some of the wellknown Boston families, and conservative tendencies in others. The traits of blood seem to outlast successive series of special reforms. Be this as it may, it is safe to assume, that, as the anti-slavery movement prevailed with only a moderate amount of sanction from "our best society," the woman-suffrage movement, which has at least an equal amount, has no reason to be discouraged.

But on looking farther, we find that not reforms alone, but often most important and established institutions, exist and flourish with only incidental aid from those "in society." Take, for instance, the whole public-school system of our larger cities. Grant that out of twenty ladies "in society," taken at random, not more than one would personally approve of women's voting: it is doubtful whether even that proportion of them would personally favor the public-school system so far as to submit their children, or at least their girls, to it. Yet the public schools flourish, and give a better training than most private schools, in spite of this inert practical resistance from those "in society." The natural inference would seem to be, that if an institution so well established as the public schools, and so generally recognized, can afford to be ignored by "society," then certainly a wholly new reform must expect no better fate.

As a matter of fact, I apprehend that what is called "society," in the sense of the more fastidious or exclusive social circle in any community, exists for one sole object,—the preservation of good manners and social refinements. For this purpose it is put very largely under the sway of women, who have, all the world over, a better instinct for these important things. It is true that "society" is apt to do even this duty very imperfectly, and often tolerates, and sometimes even cultivates, just the rudeness and discourtesy that it is set to cure. Nevertheless, this is its mission; but so soon as it steps beyond this, and attempts to claim any special weight outside the sphere of good manners, it shows its weakness, and must yield to stronger forces.

One of these stronger forces is religion, which should train men and women to a far higher standard than "society" alone can teach. This standard should be embodied, theoretically, in the Christian Church; but unhappily "society" is too often stronger than this embodiment, and turns the church itself into a mere temple of fashion. Other opposing forces are known as science and common-sense, which is only science written in short-hand. On some of these various forces all reforms are based, the woman-suffrage reform among them. If it could really be shown that some limited social circle was opposed to this, then the moral would seem to be, "So much the worse for the social circle." It used to be thought in anti-slavery days that one of the most blessed results of that agitation was the education it gave to young men and women who would otherwise have merely grown up "in society," but were happily taken in hand by a stronger influence. It is Goethe who suggests, when discussing Hamlet in "Wilhelm Meister," that, if an oak be planted in a flower-pot, it will be worse in the end for the flower-pot than for the tree. And to those who watch, year after year, the young human seedlings planted "in society," the main point of interest lies in the discovery which of these are likely to grow into oaks.

But the truth is, that the very use of the word "society" in this sense is narrow and misleading. We Americans are fortunate enough to live in a larger society, where no conventional position or family traditions exert an influence that is to be in the least degree compared with the influence secured by education, energy, and character. No matter how fastidious the social circle, one is constantly struck with the limitations of its influence, and with the little power exerted by its members as compared with that which may easily be wielded by tongue and pen. No merely fashionable woman in New York, for instance, has a position sufficiently important to be called influential compared with that of a woman who can speak in public so as to command hearers, or can write so as to secure readers. To be at the head of a normal school, or to be a professor in a college where co-education prevails, is to have a sway over the destinies of America which reduces all mere "social position" to a matter of cards and compliments and page's buttons.

XLII.
THE BATTLE OF THE CARDS.

The great winter's contest of the visiting-cards recommences at the end of every autumn. Suspended during the summer, or only renewed at Newport and such thoroughbred and thoroughly sophisticated haunts, it will set in with fury in the habitable regions of our cities once more. Now will the atmosphere around Fifth Avenue in New York be darkened—or whitened—at the appointed hour by the shower of pasteboard transmitted from dainty kid-gloved hands to the cotton-gloved hands of "John," through him to reach the possibly gloveless hands of some other John, who stands obsequious in the doorway. Now will every lady, after John has slammed the door, drive happily on to some other door, re-arranging, as she goes, her display of cards, laid as if for a game on the opposite seat of her carriage, and dealt perhaps in four suits,—her own cards, her daughters', her husband's, her "Mr. and Mrs." cards, and who knows how many more? With all this ammunition, what a very *mitrailleuse* of good society she becomes; what an accumulation of polite attentions she may discharge at any door! That one well-appointed woman, as she sits in her carriage, represents the total visiting power of self, husband, daughters, and possibly a son or two beside. She has all their counterfeit presentments in her hands. How happy she is! and how happy will the others be on her return, to think that dear mamma has disposed of so many dear, beloved, tiresome, social foes that morning! It will be three months at least, they think, before the A's and the B's and the C's will have to be "done" again.

Ah! but who knows how soon these fatiguing letters of the alphabet, rallying to the defence, will come, pasteboard in hand, to return the onset? In this contest, fair ladies, "there are blows to take, as well as blows to give," in the words of the immortal Webster. Some day, on returning, you will find a half-dozen cards on your own table that will undo all this morning's work, and send you forth on the war-path again. Is it not like a campaign? It is from this subtle military analogy, doubtless, that when gentlemen happen to quarrel, in the very best society, they exchange cards as preliminary to a duel; and that, when French journalists fight, all other French journalists show their sympathy for the survivor by sending him their cards. When we see, therefore, these heroic ladies riding forth in the social battle's magnificently stern array, our hearts render them the homage due to the brave. When we consider how complex their military equipment has grown, we fancy each of these self-devoted mothers to be an Arnold Winkelried, receiving in her martyr-breast the points of a dozen different cards, and shouting, "Make way for liberty!" For is it not securing liberty to have cleared off a dozen calls from your list, and found nobody at home?

If this sort of thing goes on, who can tell where the paper warfare shall end? If ladies may leave cards for their husbands, who are never seen out of Wall Street, except when they are seen at their clubs; or for their sons, who never forsake their billiards or their books,—why can they not also leave them for their ancestors, or for their remotest posterity? Who knows but people may yet drop cards in the names of the grandchildren whom they only wish for, or may reconcile hereditary feuds by interchanging pasteboard in behalf of two hostile grandparents who died half a century ago?

And there is another social observance in which the introduction of the card system may yet be destined to save much labor,—the attendance on fashionable churches. Already, it is said, a family may sometimes reconcile devout observance with a late breakfast, by stationing the family carriage near the church-door—empty. Really, it would not be a much emptier observance to send the cards alone by the footman; and doubtless, in the progress of civilization, we shall yet reach that point. It will have many advantages. The *effete* of society, as some cruel satirist has called them, may then send their orisons on pasteboard to as many different shrines as they approve; thus insuring their souls, as it were, at several different offices. Church architecture may be simplified, for it will require nothing but a card-basket. The clergyman will celebrate his solemn ritual, and will then look in that convenient receptacle for the names of his fellow worshippers, as a fine lady, after her "reception," looks over the cards her footman hands her, to know which of her dear friends she has been welcoming. Religion as well as social proprieties will glide smoothly over a surface of glazed pasteboard; and it will be only very humble Christians indeed who will do their worshipping in person, and will hold to the worn-out and obsolete practice of "No Cards."

XLIII.
SOME WORKING-WOMEN.

It is almost a stereotyped remark, that the women of the more fashionable and worldly class, in America, are indolent, idle, incapable, and live feeble and lazy lives. It has always seemed to me that, on the contrary, they are compelled, by the very circumstances of their situation, to lead very laborious lives, requiring great strength and energy. Whether many of their pursuits are frivolous, is a different question; but that they are arduous, I do not see how any one can doubt. I think it can be easily shown that the common charges against American fashionable women do not hold against the class I describe.

There is, for instance, the charge of evading the cares of housekeeping, and of preferring a boarding-house or hotel. But no woman with high aims in the world of fashion can afford to relieve herself from household cares in this way, except as an exceptional or occasional thing. She must keep house in order to have entertainments, to form a circle, to secure a position. The law of give and take is as absolute in society as in business; and the very first essential to social position in our larger cities is a household and a hospitality of one's own. It is far more practicable for a family of high rank in England to live temporarily in lodgings in London, than for any family with social aspirations to do the same in New York. The married woman who seeks a position in the world of society, must, therefore, keep house.

And, with housekeeping, there comes at once to the American woman a world of care far beyond that of her European sisters. Abroad, every thing in domestic life is systematized; and services of any grade, up to that of housekeeper or steward, can be secured for money, and for a moderate amount of that. The mere amount of money might not trouble the American woman; but where to get the service? Such a thing as a trained housekeeper, who can undertake, at any salary, to take the work off the shoulders of the lady of the house,—such a thing America hardly affords. Without this, the multiplication of servants only increaseth sorrow; the servants themselves are commonly an undisciplined mob, and the lady of the house is like a general attempting to drill his whole command personally, without the aid of a staff-officer or so much as a sergeant. For an occasional grand entertainment, she can, perhaps, import a special force; some fashionable sexton can arrange her invitations, and some genteel caterer her supper. But for the daily routine of the household—guests, children, door-bell, equipage—there is one vast, constant toil every day; and the woman who would have these things done well must give her own orders, and discipline her own retinue. The husband may have no "business," his wealth may supersede the necessity of all toil beyond daily billiards; but for the wife wealth means business, and, the more complete the social triumph, the more overwhelming the daily toil.

For instance, I know a fair woman in an Atlantic city who is at the head of a household including six children and nine servants. The whole domestic management is placed absolutely in her hands: she engages or dismisses every person employed, incurs every expense, makes every purchase, and keeps all the accounts; her husband only ordering the fuel, directing the affairs of the stable, and drawing checks for the bills. Every hour of her morning is systematically appropriated to these things. Among other things, she has to provide for nine meals a day; in dining-room, kitchen, and nursery, three each. Then she has to plan her social duties, and to drive out, exquisitely dressed, to make her calls. Then there are constantly dinner-parties and evening entertainments; she reads a little, and takes lessons in one or two languages. Meanwhile her husband has for daily occupation his books, his club, and the above-mentioned light and easy share in the cares of the household. Many men in his position do not even keep an account of personal expenditures.

There is nothing exceptional in this lady's case, except that the work may be better done than usual: the husband could not well contribute more than his present share without hurting domestic discipline; nor does the wife do all this from pleasure, but in a manner from necessity. It is the condition of her social position: to change it, she must withdraw herself from her social world. A few improvements, such as "family hotels," are doing something to relieve this class to whom luxury means labor. The great under-current which is sweeping us all toward some form of associated life is as obvious in this new improvement in housekeeping, as in co-operative stores or trades-unions; but it will nevertheless be long before the "women of society" in America can be any thing but a hard-working class.

The question is not whether such a life as I have described is the ideal life. My point is that it is, at any rate, a life demanding far more of energy and toil, at least in America, than the men of the same class are called upon to exhibit. There is growing up a class of men of leisure in America; but there are no women of leisure in the same circle. They hold their social position on condition of "an establishment," and an establishment makes them working-women. One result is the constant exodus of this class to Europe, where domestic life is just now easier. Another consequence is, that you hear woman suffrage denounced by women of this class, not on the ground that it involves any harder work than they already do, but on the ground that they have work enough already, and will not bear the suggestion of any more.

XLIV.
THE EMPIRE OF MANNERS.

I was present at a lively discourse, administered by a young lady just from Europe to a veteran politician. "It is of very little consequence," she said, "what kind of men you send out as foreign ministers. The thing of real importance is that they should have the right kind of wives. Any man can sign a treaty, I suppose, if you tell him what kind of treaty it must be. But all his social relations with the nations to which you send him will depend on his wife." There was some truth, certainly, in this audacious conclusion. It reminded me of the saying of a modern thinker, "The only empire freely conceded to women is that of manners—but it is worth all the rest put together."

Every one instinctively feels that the graces and amenities of life must be largely under the direction of women. The fact that this feeling has been carried too far, and has led to the dwarfing of women's intellect, must not lead to a rejection of this important social sphere. It is too strong a power to be ignored. George Eliot says well that "the commonest man, who has his ounce of sense and feeling, is conscious of the difference between a lovely, delicate woman, and a coarse one. Even a dog feels a difference in their presence." At a summer resort, for instance, one sees women who may be intellectually very ignorant and narrow, yet whose mere manners give them a social power which the highest intellects might envy. To lend joy and grace to all one's little world of friendship; to make one's house a place which every guest enters with eagerness, and leaves with reluctance; to lend encouragement to the timid, and ease to the awkward; to repress violence, restrain egotism, and make even controversy courteous,—these belong to the empire of woman. It is a sphere so important and so beautiful, that even courage and self-devotion seem not quite enough, without the addition of this supremest charm.

This courtesy is so far from implying falsehood, that its very best basis is perfect simplicity. Given a naturally sensitive organization, a loving spirit, and the early influence of a refined home, and the foundation of fine manners is secured. A person so favored may be reared in a log-hut, and may pass easily into a palace; the few needful conventionalities are so readily acquired. But I think it is a mistake to tell children, as we sometimes do, that simplicity and a kind heart are absolutely all that are needful in the way of manners. There are persons in whom simplicity and kindness are inborn, and who yet never attain to good manners for want of refined perceptions. And it is astonishing how much refinement alone can do, even if it is not very genuine or very full of heart, to smooth the paths and make social life attractive.

All the acute observers have recognized the difference between the highest standard, which is nature's, and that next to the highest, which is art's. George Eliot speaks of that fine polish which is "the expensive substitute for simplicity," and Tennyson says of manners,—

> "Kind nature's are the best: those next to best
> That fit us like a nature second-hand;
> Which are indeed the manners of the great."

In our own national history, we have learned to recognize that the personal demeanor of women may be a social and political force. The slave-power owed much of its prolonged control at Washington, and the larger part of its favor in Europe, to the fact that the manners of Southern women had been more sedulously trained than those of Northern women. Even at this moment, one may see at any watering-place that the relative social influence of different cities does not depend upon the intellectual training of their women, so much as on the manners. And, even if this is very unreasonable, the remedy would seem to be, not to go about lecturing on the intrinsic superiority of the Muses to the Graces, but to pay due homage at all the shrines.

It is a great deal to ask of reformers, especially, that they should be ornamental as well as useful; and I would by no means indorse the views of a lady who once told me that she was ready to adopt the most radical views of the women-reformers if she could see one well-dressed woman who accepted them. The place where we should draw the line between independence and deference, between essentials and non-essentials, between great ideas and little courtesies, will probably never be determined —except by actual examples. Yet it is safe to fall back on Miss Edgeworth's maxim in "Helen," that "Every one who makes goodness disagreeable commits high treason against virtue." And it is not a pleasant result of our good deeds, that others should be immediately driven into bad deeds by the burning desire to be unlike us.

XLV.
"GIRLSTEROUSNESS."

They tell the story of a little boy, a young scion of the house of Beecher, that, on being rebuked for some noisy proceeding, in which his little sister had also shared, he claimed that she also should be included in the indictment. "If a boy makes too much noise," he said, "you tell him he mustn't be boisterous. Well, then, when a girl makes just as much noise, you ought to tell her not to be *girlsterous*."

I think that we should accept, with a sense of gratitude, this addition to the language. It supplies a name for a special phase of feminine demeanor, inevitably brought out of modern womanhood. Any transitional state of society develops some evil with the good. Good results are unquestionably proceeding from the greater freedom now allowed to women. The drawback is, that we are developing, here and now, more of "girlsterousness" than is apt to be seen in less-enlightened countries.

The more complete the subjection of woman, the more "subdued" in every sense she is. The typical woman of savage life is, at least in youth, gentle, shy, retiring, timid. A Bedouin woman is modest and humble; an Indian girl has a voice "gentle and low." The utmost stretch of the imagination cannot picture either of them as "girlsterous." That perilous quality can only come as woman is educated, self-respecting, emancipated. "Girlsterousness" is the excess attendant on that virtue, the shadow which accompanies that light. It is more visible in England than in France, in America than in England.

It is to be observed, that, if a girl wishes to be noisy, she can be as noisy as anybody. Her noise, if less clamorous, is more shrill and penetrating. The shrieks of schoolgirls, playing in the yard at recess-time, seem to drown the voices of the boys. As you enter an evening party, it is the women's tones you hear most conspicuously. There is no defect in the organ, but at least an adequate vigor. In travelling by rail, when sitting near some rather under-bred party of youths and damsels, I have commonly noticed that the girls were the noisiest. The young men appeared more regardful of public opinion, and looked round with solicitude, lest they should attract too much attention. It is "girlsterousness" that dashes straight on, regardless of all observers.

Of course reformers exhibit their full share of this undesirable quality. Where the emancipation of women is much discussed in any circle, some young girls will put it in practice gracefully and with dignity, others rudely. Yet even the rudeness may be but a temporary phase, and at last end well. When women were being first trained as physicians, years ago, I remember a young girl who came from a Southern State to a Northern city, and attended the medical lectures. Having secured her lecture-tickets, she also bought season-tickets to the theatre and to the pistol-gallery, laid in a box of cigars, and began her professional training. If she meant it as a satire on the pursuits of the young gentlemen around her, it was not without point. But it was, I suppose, a clear case of "girlsterousness;" and I dare say that she sowed her wild oats much more innocently than many of her male contemporaries, and that she has long since become a sedate matron. But I certainly cannot commend her as a model.

Yet I must resolutely deny that any sort of hoydenishness or indecorum is an especial characteristic of radicals, or even "provincials," as a class. Some of the fine ladies who would be most horrified at the "girlsterousness" of this young maiden would themselves smoke their cigarettes in much worse company, morally speaking, than she ever tolerated. And, so far as manners are concerned, I am bound to say that the worst cases of rudeness and ill-breeding that have ever come to my knowledge have not occurred in the "rural districts," or among the lower ten thousand, but in those circles of America where the whole aim in life might seem to be the cultivation of its elegances.

And what confirms me in the fear that the most profound and serious types of this disease are not to be found in the wildcat regions is the fact that so much of is transplanted to Europe, among those who have the money to travel. It is there described broadly as "Americanism;" and, so surely as any peculiarly shrill group is heard coming through a European picture-gallery, it is straightway classed by all observers as belonging to the great Republic. If the observers are enamoured at sight with the beauty of the young ladies of the party, they excuse the voices;

"Strange or wild, or madly gay,
They call it only pretty Fanny's way."

But other observers are more apt to call it only Columbia's way; and if they had ever heard the word "girlsterousness," they would use that too.

Emerson says, "A gentleman makes no noise; a lady is serene." If we Americans often violate this perfect maxim of good manners, it is something that America has, at least, furnished the maxim. And, between Emerson and "girlsterousness," our courteous philosopher will yet carry the day.

XLVI.
ARE WOMEN NATURAL ARISTOCRATS?

A clergyman's wife in England has lately set on foot a reform movement in respect to dress; and, like many English reformers, she aims chiefly to elevate the morals and manners of the lower classes, without much reference to her own social equals. She proposes that "no servant, under pain of dismissal, shall wear flowers, feathers, brooches, buckles or clasps, ear-rings, lockets, neck-ribbons, velvets, kid gloves, parasols, sashes, jackets, or trimming of any kind on dresses, and, above all, no crinoline; no pads to be worn, or frisettes, or *chignons*, or hair-ribbons. The dress is to be gored and made just to touch the ground, and the hair to be drawn closely to the head, under a round white cap, without trimming of any kind. The same system of dress is recommended for Sunday-school girls, school-mistresses, church-singers, and the lower orders generally."

The remark is obvious, that in this country such a course of discipline would involve the mistress, not the maid, in the "pain of dismissal." The American clergyman and clergyman's wife who should even "recommend" such a costume to a school-mistress, church-singer, or Sunday-school girl, —to say nothing of the rest of the "lower orders,"—would soon find themselves without teachers, without pupils, without a choir, and probably without a parish. It is a comfort to think that even in older countries there is less and less of this impertinent interference: the costume of different ranks is being more and more assimilated; and the incidental episode of a few liveries in our cities is not enough to interfere with the general current. Never yet, to my knowledge, have I seen even a livery worn by a white native American; and to restrain the Sunday bonnets of her handmaidens, what lady has attempted?

This is as it should be. The Sunday bonnet of the Irish damsel is only the symbol of a very proper effort to obtain her share of all social advantages. Long may those ribbons wave! Meanwhile I think the fact that it is easier for the gentleman of the house to control the dress of his groom than for the lady to dictate that of her waiting-maid,—this must count against the theory that it is women who are the natural aristocrats.

Women are no doubt more sensitive than men upon matters of taste and breeding. This is partly from a greater average fineness of natural perception, and partly because their more secluded lives give them less of miscellaneous contact with the world. If Maud Müller and her husband had gone to board at the same boarding-house with the Judge and his wife, that lady might have held aloof from the rustic bride, simply from inexperience in life, and not knowing just how to approach her. But the Judge, who might have been talking politics or real estate with the young farmer on the doorsteps that morning, would certainly find it easier to deal with him as a man and a brother at the dinner-table. From these different causes women get the credit or discredit of being more aristocratic than men are; so that in England the Tory supporters of female suffrage base it on the ground that these new voters at least will be conservative.

But, on the other hand, it is women, even more than men, who are attracted by those strong qualities of personal character which are always the antidote to aristocracy. No bold revolutionist ever defied the established conventionalisms of his times without drawing his strongest support from women. Poet and novelist love to depict the princess as won by the outlaw, the gypsy, the peasant. Women have a way of turning from the insipidities and proprieties of life to the wooer who has the stronger hand; from the silken Darnley to the rude Bothwell. This impulse is the natural corrective to the aristocratic instincts of womanhood; and though men feel it less, it is still, even among them, one of the supports of republican institutions. We need to keep always balanced between the two influences of refined culture and of native force. The patrician class, wherever there is one, is pretty sure to be the more refined; the plebeian class, the more energetic. That woman is able to appreciate both elements, is proof that she is quite capable of doing her share in social and political life. This English clergyman's wife, who devotes her soul to the trimmings and gored skirts of the lower orders, is no more entitled to represent her sex than are those ladies who give their whole attention to the "novel and intricate bonnets" advertised this season on Broadway.

XLVII.
MRS. BLANK'S DAUGHTERS.

Mrs. Blank, of Far West—let us not draw her from the "sacred privacy of woman" by giving the name or place too precisely—has an insurmountable objection to woman's voting. So the newspapers say; and this objection is, that she does not wish her daughters to encounter disreputable characters at the polls.

It is a laudable desire, to keep one's daughters from the slightest contact with such persons. But how does Mrs. Blank precisely mean to accomplish this? Will she shut up the maidens in a harem? When they go out, will she send messengers through the streets to bid people hide their faces, as when an Oriental queen is passing? Will she send them travelling on camels, veiled by *yashmaks*? Will she prohibit them from being so much as seen by a man, except when a physician must be called for their ailments, and Miss Blank puts her arm through a curtain, in order that he may feel her pulse and know no more?

Who is Mrs. Blank, and how does she bring up her daughters? Does she send them to the post-office? If so, they may wait a half-hour at a time for the mail to open, and be elbowed by the most disreputable characters, waiting at their side. If it does the young ladies no harm to encounter this for the sake of getting their letters out, will it harm them to do it in order to get their ballots in? If they go to hear Gough lecture, they may be kept half an hour at the door, elbowed by saint and sinner indiscriminately. If it is worth going through this to hear about temperance, why not to vote about it? If they go to Washington to the President's inauguration, they may stand two hours with Mary Magdalen on one side of them and Judas Iscariot on the other. If this contact is rendered harmless by the fact that they are receiving political information, will it hurt them to stay five minutes longer in order to act upon the knowledge they have received?

This is on the supposition that the household of Blank are plain, practical women, unversed in the vanities of the world. If they belong to fashionable circles, how much harder to keep them wholly clear of disreputable contact! Should they, for instance, visit Newport, they may possibly be seen at the Casino, looking very happy as they revolve rapidly in the arms of some very disreputable characters; they will be seen in the surf, attired in the most scanty and clinging drapery, and kindly aided to preserve their balance by the devoted attentions of the same companions. Mrs. Blank, meanwhile, will look complacently on, with the other matrons: they are not supposed to know the current reputation of those whom their daughters meet "in society;" and, so long as there is no actual harm done, why should they care? Very well; but why, then, should they care if they encounter those same disreputable characters when they go to drop a ballot in the ballot-box? It will be a more guarded and distant meeting. It is not usual to dance round-dances at the ward-room, so far as I know, or to bathe in clinging drapery at that rather dry and dusty resort. If such very close intimacies are all right under the gas-light or at the beach, why should there be poison in merely passing a disreputable character at the City Hall?

On the whole, the prospects of Mrs. Blank are not encouraging. Should she consult a physician for her daughters, he may be secretly or openly disreputable; should she call in a clergyman, he may, though a bishop, have carnal rather than spiritual eyes. If Miss Blank be caught in a shower, she may take refuge under the umbrella of an undesirable acquaintance; should she fall on the ice, the woman who helps to raise her may have sinned. There is not a spot in any known land where a woman can live in absolute seclusion from all contact with evil. Should the Misses Blank even turn Roman Catholics, and take to a convent, their very confessor may be secretly a scoundrel; and they may be glad to flee for refuge to the busy, buying, selling, dancing, voting world outside.

No: Mrs. Blank's prayers for absolute protection will never be answered, in respect to her daughters. Why not, then, find a better model for prayer in that made by Jesus for his disciples: "I pray Thee, not that Thou shouldst take them out of the world, but that Thou shouldst keep them from the evil." A woman was made for something nobler in the world, Mrs. Blank, than to be a fragile toy, to be put behind a glass case, and protected from contact. It is not her mission to be hidden away from all life's evil, but bravely to work that the world may be reformed.

XLVIII.
THE EUROPEAN PLAN.

Every mishap among American women brings out renewed suggestions of what maybe called the "European plan" in the training of young girls,—the plan, that is, of extreme seclusion and helplessness. It is usually forgotten, in these suggestions, that not much protection is really given anywhere to this particular class as a whole. Everywhere in Europe, the restrictions are of caste, not of sex. Even in Turkey, travellers tell us, women of the humbler vocations are not much secluded. It is not the object of the "European plan," in any form, to protect the virtue of young women, as such, but only of young ladies; and the protection is pretty effectually limited to that order. Among the Portuguese, in the island of Fayal, I found it to be the ambition of each humble family to bring up one daughter in a sort of ladylike seclusion: she never went into the street alone, or without a hood which was equivalent to a veil; she was taught indoor industries only; she was constantly under the eye of her mother. But, in order that one daughter might be thus protected, all the other daughters were allowed to go alone, day or evening, bare-headed or bare-footed, by the loneliest mountain-paths, to bring oranges or firewood or whatever their work may be—heedless of protection. The safeguard was for a class: the average exposure of young womanhood was far greater than with us. So in London, while you rarely see a young lady alone in the streets, the housemaid is sent on errands at any hour of the evening with a freedom at which our city domestics would quite rebel; and one has to stay but a short time in Paris to see how entirely limited to a class is the alleged restraint under which young French girls are said to be kept.

Again, it is to be remembered that the whole "European plan," so far as it is applied on the Continent of Europe, is a plan based upon utter distrust and suspicion, not only as to chastity, but as to all other virtues. It is applied among the higher classes almost as consistently to boys as to girls. In every school under church auspices, it is the French theory that boys are never to be left unwatched for a moment; and it is as steadily assumed that girls will be untruthful if left to themselves, as that they will do every other wrong. This to the Anglo-Saxon race seems very demoralizing. "Suspicion," said Sir Philip Sidney, "is the way to lose that which we fear to lose." Readers of the Brontë novels will remember the disgust of the English pupils and teachers in French schools at the constant espionage around them; and I have more than once heard young girls who had been trained at such institutions say that it was a wonder if they had any truthfulness left, so invariable was the assumption that it was the nature of young girls to lie. I cannot imagine any thing less likely to create upright and noble character, in man or woman, than the systematic application of the "European plan."

And that it produces just the results that might be feared, the whole tone of European literature proves. Foreigners, no doubt, do habitual injustice to the morality of French households; but it is impossible that fiction can utterly misrepresent the community which produces and reads it. When one thinks of the utter lightness of tone with which breaches, both of truth and chastity, are treated even, in the better class of French novels and plays, it seems absurd to deny the correctness of the picture. Besides, it is not merely a question of plays and novels. Consider, for instance, the contempt with which Taine treats Thackeray for representing the mother of Pendennis as suffering agonies when she thinks that her son has seduced a young girl, his social inferior. Thackeray is not really considered a model of elevated tone, as to such matters, among English writers; but the Frenchman is simply amazed that the Englishman should describe even the saintliest of mothers as attaching so much weight to such a small affair.

An able newspaper writer, quoted with apparent approval by the Boston Daily Advertiser, praises the supposed foreign method for the "habit of dependence and deference" that it produces; and because it gives to a young man a wife whose "habit of deference is established." But it must be remembered, that, where this theory is established, the habit of deference is logically carried much farther than mere conjugal convenience would take it. Its natural outcome is the authority of the priest, not of the husband. That domination of the women of France by the priesthood which forms to-day the chief peril of the republic,—which is the strength of legitimism and imperialism and all other conspiracies against the liberty of the French people,—is only the visible and inevitable result of this dangerous docility.

One thing is certain, that the best preparation for freedom is freedom; and that no young girls are so poorly prepared for American life as those whose early years are passed in Europe. The worst imprudences, the most unmaidenly and offensive actions, that I have ever heard of in decent society, have been on the part of young women educated in Europe, who have been launched into American life without its early training,—have been treated as children until they suddenly awakened to the freedom of women. On the other hand, I remember with pleasure, that a cultivated French mother, whose daughter's fine qualities were the best seal of her motherhood, once told me that the models she had chosen in her daughter's training were certain families of American young ladies, of whom she had, through peculiar circumstances, seen much in Paris.

XLIX.
"FEATHERSES."

One of the most amusing letters ever quoted in any book is that given in Curzon's "Monasteries of the Levant," as the production of a Turkish sultana who had just learned English. It is as follows:—

Note from Adile Sultana, the betrothed of Abbas Pasha, to her Armenian Commissioner.

Constantinople, 1844.

My Noble Friend:—Here are the featherses sent my soul, my noble friend, are there no other featherses leaved in the shop beside these featherses? and these featherses remains, and these featherses are ukly. They are very dear, who buyses dheses? And my noble friend, we want a noat from yorself; those you brought last tim, those you sees were very beautiful; we had searched; my soul, I want featherses again, of those featherses. In Kalada there is plenty of feather. Whatever bees, I only want beautiful featherses; I want featherses of every desolation to-morrow.

(Signed)

You Know Who.

The first steps in culture do not, then, it seems, remove from the feminine soul the love of finery. Nor do the later steps wholly extinguish it; for did not Grace Greenwood hear the learned Mary Somerville conferring with the wise Harriet Martineau as to whether a certain dress should be dyed to match a certain shawl? Well! why not? Because women learn the use of the quill, are they to ignore "featherses"? Because they learn science, must they unlearn the arts, and above all the art of being beautiful? If men have lost it, they have reason to regret the loss. Let women hold to it, while yet within their reach.

Mrs. Rachel Howland of New Bedford, much prized and trusted as a public speaker among Friends, and a model of taste and quiet beauty in costume, delighted the young girls at a Newport Yearly Meeting, a few years since, by boldly declaring that she thought God meant women to make the world beautiful, as much as flowers and butterflies, and that there was no sin in tasteful dress, but only in devoting to it too much money or too much time. It is a blessed doctrine. The utmost extremes of dress, the love of colors, of fabrics, of jewels, of "featherses," are, after all, but an effort after the beautiful. The reason why the beautiful is not always the result is because so many women are ignorant or merely imitative. They have no sense of fitness: the short wear what belongs to the tall, and brunettes sacrifice their natural beauty to look like blondes. Or they have no adaptation; and even an emancipated woman may show a disregard for appropriateness, as where a fine lady sweeps the streets, or a fair orator the platform, with a silken or velvet train which accords only with a carpet as luxurious as itself. What is inappropriate is never beautiful. What is merely in the fashion is never beautiful. But who does not know some woman whose taste and training are so perfect that fashion becomes to her a means of grace instead of a despot, and the worst excrescence that can be prescribed—a *chignon*, a hoop, a panier—is softened into something so becoming that even the Parisian bondage seems but a chain of roses?

In such hands, even "featherses" become a fine art, not a matter of vanity. Are women so much more vain than men? No doubt they talk more about their dress, for there is much more to talk about; yet did you never hear the men of fashion discuss boots and hats and the liveries of grooms? A good friend of mine, a shoemaker, who supplies very high heels for a great many pretty feet on Fifth Avenue in New York, declares that women are not so vain of their feet as men. "A man who thinks he has a handsome foot," quoth our fashionable Crispin, "is apt to give us more trouble than any lady among our customers. I have noticed this for twenty years." The testimony is consoling—to women.

And this naturally suggests the question, What is to be the future of masculine costume? Is the present formlessness and gracelessness and monotony of hue to last forever, as suited to the rough needs of a work-a-day world? It is to be remembered that the difference in this respect between the dress of the sexes is a very recent thing. Till within a century or so men dressed as picturesquely as women, and paid as minute attention to their costume. Even the fashions in armor varied as extensively as the fashions in gowns. One of Henry III.'s courtiers, Sir J. Arundel, had fifty-two complete suits of cloth of gold. No satin, no velvet, was too elegant for those who sat to Copley for their pictures. In Puritan days the laws could hardly be made severe enough to prevent men from wearing silver-lace and "broad bone-lace," and shoulder-bands of undue width, and double ruffs and "immoderate great breeches." What seemed to the Cavaliers the extreme of stupid sobriety in dress, would pass now for the most fantastic array. Fancy Samuel Pepys going to a wedding of to-day in his "new colored silk suit and coat trimmed with gold buttons, and gold broad lace round his hands, very rich and fine." It would give to the ceremony the aspect of a fancy ball; yet how much prettier a sight is a fancy ball than the ordinary entertainment of the period!

Within the last few years the rigor of masculine costume is a little relaxed; velvets are resuming their picturesque sway: and, instead of the customary suit of solemn black, gentlemen are appearing in blue and gold editions at evening parties. Let us hope that good sense and taste may yet meet each other, for both sexes; that men may borrow for their dress some womanly taste, women some masculine sense; and society may again witness a graceful and appropriate costume, without being too much absorbed in "featherses."

L.
SOME MAN-MILLINERY.

We may breathe more freely. The religious prospects of America brighten. Our dealers have received the "Catalogue of Clerical Vestments and Improved Church Ornaments manufactured by Simon Jeune, 34 Rue de Cléry, Paris."

Why are we not a nation of saints? Plainly, because the church-apparatus has hitherto been so very deficient. Religion has been, so to speak, naked. The dry-goods stores, supplying only the laity, have left the clergy unclothed. In what ready-made-clothing store can you find any thing like a proper alb? Ask your tailor, if you dare, for a chasuble. At Stewart's shop New Yorkers boast that you can buy any thing; but fancy a respectable citizen entering those marble portals, and demanding a cope or a dalmatic! As for an ombrellino, or an antependium, you might as well attempt to go buffalo-hunting in Broadway. In that case you would at least find the dried skin of the animal; but we doubt if there is to be found on sale any thing nearer an ombrellino than a lady's parasol. They order this thing otherwise in France.

Mr. Simon Jeune provides every one of these simple luxuries. Not a device by which a rich man may enter the kingdom of heaven, but he has it at his fingers' ends. None of your cheap salvations mar the dignity of 34 Rue de Cléry. "We do not manufacture these articles at a low price," he calmly announces. There is no limit in the other direction. You can lead souls to heaven in a robe worth twenty-five guineas; but, if you insist on parsimony in your piety, you must patronize some other establishment.

Yet who that reads this catalogue, and revels for a half-hour amid its gold and jewels, would care to be parsimonious? What is money worth, except as a means of putting one's favorite minister into a chasuble "in gold cloth with glazed friz ground, double superior quality"? Since the Christian must at any rate bear his cross, is it not a satisfaction to have it "on a gold ground, richly worked in gold and silver"? If there is no true religion without a cope, is it not well that its "hood and orfraies" should be "surrounded with glazed gold-columned galloon"? And, as death must come at any rate, is it not something that your pall may bear "a handsome design of silver tears in emboss in the centre of the cross," price only six guineas?

Time would fail to tell of the banners and the dais, the altar-cloths and frontals, the pastoral stoles and benediction-scarfs, the pyxes and chalices, and, in short, all dear delights of consecrated souls. This saintly upholsterer makes as many "fresh sacrifices," it would appear, as any other retailer; but, as this does not prevent him from pricing a dais as high as four hundred pounds sterling, there is no danger of the purchasers finding any thing cheap enough to be really discreditable. And the goods are all warranted to be as indestructible as the lowly virtues they symbolize.

M. Jeune positively announces that he "supplies every article connected with the Roman Catholic Church." Perhaps he reserves the faith, hope, and charity for the next catalogue, as they do not appear largely in this. In other respects, reading this catalogue is as good as a seat in the most fashionable church, and leaves much the same impression. It is especially useful for summer-time, when one may wander in the country, to the peril of one's soul, and may consider the lilies a great deal too much, and may come to thinking religion a thing obtainable on cheap terms, after all. This would not do for M. Jeune's business: let us return to the realities of time and eternity, and consider this "embroidered glory of spangles and prul,"— whatever prul may be.

But can it, after all, be possible that these gorgeous garments are to be worn by men only, and that those same men will sometimes treat it as a reproach to women that they are fond of dress?

LI.
SUBLIME PRINCES IN DISTRESS.

In looking over some miscellaneous papers which came, the other day, into my hands, I found among them a newspaper scrap, expressing certain criticisms familiar to the inquiring mind. It stated the predominant attribute of women to be frivolity; an inordinate love of show, display, rank, title, dress; a habit of absorption in the petty details of these follies, to the exclusion of all serious thought and purpose. In reading this lucubration, one was led to suppose that the whole aim of all women was to meet in little circles where they could wear costly attire, call themselves by fine names, and, in the concise Italian phrase, "peacock themselves" generally.

But there happened to be among the same papers another class of documents which tended to unsettle the mind a little on these topics. These documents were in print, and were not marked as private, or addressed to any particular name, so that there can be no harm in reprinting one of them, suppressing, however, all reference to particular persons or places, lest I should be innocently betraying some awful secret. The paper affording most information was as follows, the dashes of omission (——) being mine, but all the rest being given *verbatim*:—

"Lux e tenebris."

—— CONSISTORY.

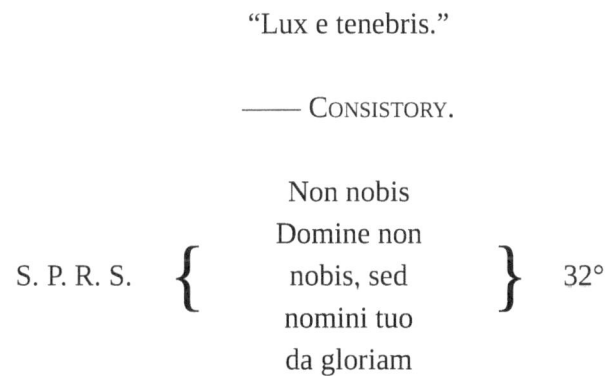

Sublime Prince:

A stated rendezvous of —— Consistory, A. A. S. Rite, will be held on the 15th day of the month Adar, A. H. 5640, in —— Hall, under the c. c. of the 3, near the B. B. at Five o'clock P.M.

Per order of

———— ————

Ill. Com. in Chief.

Ill. Grand Secretary.

The object of this meeting is thus stated: "Work: the grade of Knight Kadosh, the 30th, will be worked in full at this Rendezvous." And it appears that this work must have something of a military character; for it seems from another circular, which I will not quote in full, that the purpose of the rendezvous can be much better carried out if the members will provide themselves with a costly uniform, including a sword and other equipments. Yet it would also appear that the expenses of this organization, apart from the uniform, are so great as to call forth the following notice:—

"Delinquents.—The Finance Committee recommend the discharge from Membership of the following Sublime Princes, for non-payment of dues, they having failed to make any satisfactory reply to repealed notices of their indebtedness." [Then follows a list of names and amounts varying from $17 to $23.]

One of the most brilliant of recent French novels, Daudet's "Les Rois en Exil," lays its whole plot among the forlorn class of dethroned sovereigns in Paris; but really their sorrows do not touch an American heart so deeply as this black-list. Here are nearly twenty Princes on our own soil who are publicly exposed in a single circular as refusing, after "repeated notices of their indebtedness," even to reply satisfactorily. What pleasure can there be in the most attractive "rendezvous," what joy in the most absorbing "work," when one thinks of all these fallen Sublime Princes wandering, like Milton's angels, into outer darkness? I almost blush to own that I recognize among the names of these outcasts one or two acquaintances of my own, who certainly passed for honest men before they became princes.

But the most interesting question for women to consider is this: Who conducts this picturesque consistory, with its rites, its titles, and its uniforms? Which sex is it that makes up this society, and twenty other societies so absorbing in their "work" that some worthy persons have a "society" for almost every evening in the week? Is it the sex which is alleged to be frivolous, dressy, and eager for rank and title? Or is it the grave sex, the serious and hard-working sex, the "noble sex," *le sexe noble*, as some of the French grammars call it? No doubt there is under all this display and formality, in this "consistory," as in most similar organizations, a great deal of mutual help and friendliness. But so there is under even the seeming frivolities of women: the majority of fashionable women have good hearts, and do good. If substantial and practical men like to cover even their benevolent organizations with something of show and display, and to "peacock themselves" a little, why should not women be permitted the same privilege? Surely Sublime Princes should stand by their order, and not look with disdain on those who would like to be Sublime Princesses if they only could.

EDUCATION.

"Movet me ingens scientiarum admiratio, seu legis communis æquitas, ut in nostro sexu, rarum non esse feram, id quod omnium votis dignissimum est. Nam cum sapientia tantum generis humani ornamentum sit, ut ad omnes et singulos (quoad quidem per sortem cujusque liceat) extendi jure debeat, non vidi, cur virgini, in qua excolendi sese ornandique sedulitatem admittimus, non conveniat mundus hic omnium longè pulcherrimus."—Annæ Mariæ À Schurman Epistolæ. (1638.)

"A great reverence for knowledge and the natural sense of justice urge me to encourage in my own sex that which is most worthy the aspirations of all. For, since wisdom is so great an ornament of the human race that it should of right be extended (so far as practicable) to each and every one, I did not see why this fairest of ornaments should not be appropriate for the maiden, to whom we permit all diligence in the decoration and adornment of herself."

LII.
"EXPERIMENTS."

Why is it, that, whenever any thing is done for women in the way of education, it is called "an experiment,"—something that is to be long considered, stoutly opposed, grudgingly yielded, and dubiously watched,—while, if the same thing is done for men, its desirableness is assumed as a matter of course, and the thing is done? Thus, when Harvard College was founded, it was not regarded as an experiment, but as an institution. The "General Court," in 1636, "agreed to give 400*l*. towards a schoale or colledge," and the affair was settled. Every subsequent step in the expanding of educational opportunities for young men has gone in the same way. But when there seems a chance of extending, however irregularly, some of the same collegiate advantages to women, I observe that the Boston Daily Advertiser and the Atlantic Monthly, in all good faith, speak of the measure as an "experiment."

It seems to me no more of an "experiment" than when a boy who has hitherto eaten up his whole apple becomes a little touched with a sense of justice, and finally decides to offer his sister the smaller half. If he has ever regarded that offer as an experiment, the first actual trial will put the result into the list of certainties; and it will become an axiom in his mind that girls like apples. Whatever may be said about the position of women in law and society, it is clear that their educational disadvantages have been a prolonged disgrace to the other sex, and one for which women themselves are in no way accountable. When Françoise de Saintonges, in the sixteenth century, wished to establish girls' schools in France, she was hooted in the streets, and her father called together four doctors of law to decide whether she was possessed of a devil in planning to teach women, *"pour s'assurer qu'instruire des femmes n'était pas un œuvre du démon."* From that day to this, we have seen women almost always more ready to be taught than was any one else to teach them. Talk as you please about their wishing or not wishing to vote: they have certainly wished for instruction, and have had it doled out to them almost as grudgingly as if it were the ballot itself.

Consider the educational history of Massachusetts, for instance. The wife of President John Adams was born in 1744; and she says of her youth that "female education, in the best families, went no farther than writing and arithmetic." Barry tells us in his History of Massachusetts, that the public education was first provided for boys only; "but light soon broke in, and girls were allowed to attend the public schools two hours a day."[10] It appears from President Quincy's "Municipal History of Boston,"[11] that from 1790 girls were there admitted to such schools, but during the summer months only, when there were not boys enough to fill them,—from April 20 to Oct. 20 of each year. This lasted until 1822, when Boston became a city. Four years after, an attempt was made to establish a high school for girls, which was not, however, to teach Latin and Greek. It had, in the words of the school committee of 1854, "an alarming success;" and the school was abolished after eighteen months' trial, because the girls crowded into it; and as Mr. Quincy, with exquisite simplicity, records, "not one voluntarily quitted it, and there was no reason to suppose that any one admitted to the school would voluntarily quit for the whole three years, except in case of marriage!"

10. III., 323.

11. p. 21.

How amusing seems it now to read of such an "experiment" as this, abandoned only because of its overwhelming success! How absurd now seem the discussions of a few years ago!—the doubts whether young women really desired higher education, whether they were capable of it, whether their health would bear it, whether their parents would permit it. The address I gave before the Social Science Association on this subject, at Boston, May 14, 1873, now seems to me such a collection of platitudes that I hardly see how I dared come before an intelligent audience with such needless reasonings. It is as if I had soberly labored to prove that two and two make four, or that ginger is "hot i' the mouth." Yet the subsequent discussion in that meeting showed that around even these harmless and commonplace propositions the battle of debate could rage hot; and it really seemed as if even to teach women the alphabet ought still to be mentioned as "a promising experiment." Now, with the successes before us of Vassar and Wellesley and Smith Colleges, of Michigan and Cornell and Boston Universities; with the spectacle at Cambridge of young women actually reading Plato "at sight" with Professor Goodwin,—it surely seems as if the higher education of women might be considered quite beyond the stage of experiment, and might henceforth be provided for in the same common-sense and matter-of-course way which we provide for the education of young men.

And, if this point is already reached in education, how long before it will also be reached in political life, and women's voting be viewed as a matter of course, and a thing no longer experimental?

LIII.
INTELLECTUAL CINDERELLAS.

When, some thirty years ago, the extraordinary young mathematician, Truman Henry Safford, first attracted the attention of New England by his rare powers, I well remember the pains that were taken to place him under instruction by the ablest Harvard professors: the greater his abilities, the more needful that he should have careful and symmetrical training. The men of science did not say, "Stand off! let him alone! let him strive patiently until he has achieved something positively valuable, and he may be sure of prompt and generous recognition—when he is fifty years old." If such a course would have been mistaken and ungenerous if applied to Professor Safford, why is it not something to be regretted that it was applied to Mrs. Somerville? In her case, the mischief was done: she was, happily, strong enough to bear it; but, as the English critics say, we never shall know what science has lost by it. We can do nothing for her now; but we could do something for future women like her, by pointing this obvious moral for their benefit, instead of being content with a mere tardy recognition of success, after a woman has expended half a century in struggle.

It is commonly considered to be a step forward in civilization, that whereas ancient and barbarous nations exposed children to special hardships, in order to kill off the weak and toughen the strong, modern nations aim to rear all alike carefully, without either sacrificing or enfeebling. If we apply this to muscle, why not to mind? and, if to men's minds, why not to women's? Why use for men's intellects, which are claimed to be stronger, the forcing process,—offering, for instance, many thousand dollars a year in gratuities at Harvard College, that young men may be induced to come and learn,—and only withhold assistance from the weaker minds of women? A little schoolgirl once told me that she did not object to her teacher's showing partiality, but thought she "ought to show partiality to all alike." If all our university systems are wrong, and the proper diet for mathematical genius consists of fifty years' snubbing, let us employ it, by all means; but let it be applied to both sexes.

That it is the duty of women, even under disadvantageous circumstances, to prove their purpose by labor, to "verify their credentials," is true enough; but this moral is only part of the moral of Mrs. Somerville's book, and is cruelly incomplete without the other half. What a garden of roses was Mrs. Somerville's life, according to some comfortable critics! "All that for which too many women nowadays are content to sit and whine, or fitfully and carelessly struggle, came naturally and quietly to Mrs. Somerville. And the reason was, that she never asked for any thing until she had earned it; or, rather, she never asked at all, but was content to earn." Naturally and quietly! You might as well say that Garrison fought slavery "quietly," or that Frederick Douglass's escape came to him "naturally." Turn to the book itself, and see with what strong, though never bitter, feeling, the author looks back upon her hard struggle.

"I was intensely ambitious to excel in something; for I felt in my own breast that women were capable of taking a higher place in creation than that assigned them in my early days, which was very low" (p. 60). "Nor ... should I have had courage to ask any of them a question, for I should have been laughed at. I was often very sad and forlorn; not a hand held out to help me" (p. 47). "My father came home for a short time, and, somehow or other finding out what I was about, said to my mother, 'Peg, we must put a stop to this, or we shall have Mary in a strait-jacket one of these days'" (p. 54). "I continued my mathematical and other pursuits, but under great disadvantages; for, although my husband did not prevent me from studying, I met with no sympathy whatever from him, as he had a very low opinion of the capacity of my sex, and had neither knowledge of nor interest in science of any kind" (p. 57). "I was considered eccentric and foolish; and my conduct was highly disapproved of by many, especially by some members of my own family" (p. 80). "A man can always command his time under the plea of business: a woman is not allowed any such excuse" (p. 164). And so on.

At last in 1831—Mrs. Somerville being then fifty-one—her work on "The Mechanism of the Heavens" appeared. Then came universal recognition, generous if not prompt, a tardy acknowledgment. "Our relations," she says, "and others who had so severely criticised and ridiculed me, astonished at my success, were now loud in my praise."[12] No doubt. So were, probably, Cinderella's sisters loud in her praise, when the prince at last took her from the chimney-corner, and married her. They had kept for themselves, to be sure, as long as they could, the delights and opportunities of life; while she had taken the place assigned her in her early days,—"which was very low," as Mrs. Somerville says. But, for all that, they were very kind to her in the days of her prosperity; and no doubt packed their little trunks, and came to visit their dear sister at the palace, as often as she could wish. And, doubtless, the Fairyland Monthly of that day, when it came to review Cinderella's "Personal Recollections," pointed out, that, as soon as that distinguished lady had "achieved something positively valuable," she received "prompt and generous recognition."

12. p. 176.

LIV.
FOREIGN EDUCATION.

There is a fashionable phrase which always awakens my inward protest,—"the advantages of foreign education." Every summer brings within my view a large class of people who have perhaps spent their youth in Europe, and then have taken Europe for their wedding-tour; and then, after a year or two at home, have found it an excellent reason for going abroad again "to give the children the advantage of foreign education, you know." And, as it is in regard to girls that this advantage is especially claimed, it is in respect to them that I wish to speak.

In some ways, undoubtedly, the early foreign training offers an advantage. It is a thing of very great convenience to have the easy colloquial command of one or two languages beside one's own; and this can no doubt be obtained far more readily by a few years of early life abroad than by any method employed in later years at home. There are also some unquestionable advantages in respect to music, art, and European geography and history. The trouble is, that, when we have enumerated these advantages, we have mentioned all.

And, as a further trouble, it comes about that these things, being all that are better learned in Europe, are easily assumed, by what may be called our Europeanized classes, to be all that are worth learning, especially for girls. When, in such circles, you hear of a young lady as "splendidly educated," it commonly turns out that she speaks several languages admirably, and plays well on the piano, or sketches well. It is not needful for such an indorsement that she should have the slightest knowledge of mathematics, of logic, of rhetoric, of metaphysics, of political economy, of physiology, of any branch of natural science, or of any language, or literature, or history, except those of modern Europe. All these missing branches she would have been far more likely to study, if she had never been abroad: all these, or a sufficient number of them, she would have been pretty sure to study at a first-class American "academy" or high school. But all these she is almost sure to have missed in Europe,—missed them so thoroughly, indeed, that she is likely to regard with suspicion any one who knows any thing about them, as being "awfully learned."

Yet it needs no argument to show that the studies thus omitted by girls taught in Europe are the studies which train the intellect. That a girl should know her own powers of body and mind, should know how to observe, how to combine, how to think; that she should know the history and literature of the world at large, and in particular of the country in which she is to live,— this is certainly more important than that she should be able to speak two or three languages as well as a European courier, and should have nothing to say in any of them.

A very few persons I have known who contrived, while living abroad, to keep a home atmosphere round their children, and who, by great personal effort, succeeded in giving to their girls that solid early training which is to be had in every high school in this country, but is only to be obtained by personal effort, and under great disadvantages, in Europe. Wiser still, in my judgment, were those who trusted America for the main training, but contrived early to secure for their children the needful year or two of foreign life, for the learning of languages alone. Perhaps we exaggerate, too, the absolute necessity of foreign study, even for modern languages. The Russians, who are the best linguists in Europe, are not in the habit of expatriating themselves for that purpose; and perhaps we have something to learn from them in this direction, as well as in the line of Professor Runkle's machine-shops.

LV.
TEACHING THE TEACHERS.

Cotton Mather says of his father, Increase Mather, that, when he became president of Harvard College, it was from the desire to teach those who were to teach others, or, as he expresses it, not to shape the building but the builders,—*non lapides dolare sed architectos*. It is curious to see that women are admitted more readily to this higher work than to the lower. Thus I know a lady who teaches elocution professionally, and has clerical pupils among others. One of these assures me that he finds his power and influence in the pulpit much increased through her instruction. Yet there is scarcely a denomination which would admit her into the pulpit: she can direct the builders, but can take no share in the building.

It sometimes occurred to me, when a member of the legislature of Massachusetts, that the little I knew of political economy was mainly due to the assiduous reading, in childhood, of Miss Martineau's stories founded on that science. Yet it would have been thought something very astounding, were some such woman to have a seat in that legislature. So I have seen classes of young men and maidens, in a high school, reciting political economy out of Mrs. Fawcett's excellent textbook,—and sometimes reciting it to a woman; and yet, should any one of these boys ever become a member of "the Great and General Court," as the legislature is called in Massachusetts, he could not even invite this teacher, or Mrs. Fawcett herself, to sit beside him and aid him with her advice. Can any one help seeing that this distinction is a merely traditional thing, and one that cannot last?

At the last teachers' convention which I attended, I heard a lady, Mrs. Knox, give an address on the best way of teaching English composition. There was assembled a great body of teachers, some five or six hundred; the church was crowded; and yet this lady faced the audience for some three-quarters of an hour,—she being armed only with a piece of chalk and a blackboard,—and held it in close attention. Without perceptible effort, and without a word or an attitude that was otherwise than womanly and graceful, she taught the teachers, men and women alike. I do not see how it is possible that the alleged supremacy of man can long withstand such influences.

It seems very appropriate to read from town after town, in reference to the late school elections, "The first lady to deposit her ballot was Miss ———, a teacher in the high school." Who else should be first? I do not think that men generally comprehend how absurd it is to an experienced teacher, who has for years been putting into the brains of dull boys all the activity they possess, to see those boys grow up to be men and voters, and decide what to do with the money she pays in taxes, while she is set aside as "only a woman." Her pupils cannot make a speech in town-meeting, they cannot present a report on any subject, they cannot show any capacity of leadership, without exhibiting the influence she has had over them. Yet they are now as entirely beyond her direct reach as if she were a hen who had hatched ducklings, and had lived to see them swimming away. But the teachers are worse off than the hens; because they have actually taught their ducklings to swim, and could swim themselves if permitted. After all, Horace Mann builded better than he knew. Every step in the training of women as teachers implies a farther step.

LVI.
"CUPID-AND-PSYCHOLOGY."

The learned Master of Trinity College, Cambridge, England, is frequently facetious; and his jokes are quoted with the deference due to the chief officer of the chief college of that great university. Now, it is known that the Cambridge colleges, and Trinity College in particular, are doing a great deal for the instruction of women. The young women of Girton College and Newnham College,—both of these being institutions for women, in or near Cambridge,—not only enjoy the instruction of the university, but they share it under a guaranty that it shall be of the best quality; because they attend, in many cases, the very same lectures with the young men. Where this is not done, they sometimes use the vacant lecture-rooms of the college; and it was in connection with an application for this privilege that the Master of Trinity College made his last joke,—the last, at any rate, that has crossed the Atlantic. When told that the lecture-room was needed for a class of young women in psychology, he said, "Psychology? What kind of psychology? Cupid-and-Psychology, I suppose."

Cupid-and-Psychology is, after all, not so bad a department of instruction. It may be taken as a good enough symbol of that mingling of head and heart which is the best result of all training. One of the worst evils of the separate education of the sexes has been the easy assumption that men were to be made all head, and women all heart. It was to correct the evils of this, that Ben Jonson proposed for his ideal woman

> "a learned and a manly soul."

It was an implied recognition of it from the other side when the great masculine intellect, Goethe, held up as a guiding force in his Faust "the eternal womanly" (*das ewige weibliche*). After all, each sex must teach the other, and impart to the other. It will never do to have all the brains poured into one human being, and christened "man;" and all the affections decanted into another, and labelled "woman." Nature herself rejects this theory. Darwin himself, the interpreter of nature, shows that there is a perpetual effort going on, by unseen forces, to equalize the sexes, since sons often inherit from the mother, and daughters from the father. And we all take pleasure in discovering in the noblest of each sex something of the qualities of the other,—the tender affections in great men, the imperial intellect in great women.

On the whole, there is no harm, but rather good, in the new science of Cupid-and-Psychology. There are combinations for which no single word can suffice. The phrase belongs to the same class with Lowell's witty denunciation of a certain tiresome letter-writer, as being, not his incubus, but his "pen-and-inkubus." It is as well to admit it first as last: Cupid-and-Psychology will be taught wherever young men and women study together. Not in the direct and simple form of mutual love-making, perhaps; for they tell the visitor, at universities which admit both sexes, that the young men and maidens do not fall in love with each other, but are apt to seek their mates elsewhere. The new science has a wider bearing, and suggests that the brain is incomplete, after all, without the affections; and so are the affections without the brain. The very professorship at Harvard University which Rev. Dr. Peabody is just leaving, and which Rev. Phillips Brooks has been invited to fill, was founded by a woman, Miss Plummer; and the name proposed by her for it was "a professorship of the heart," though they after all called it only a professorship of "Christian morals." We need the heart in our colleges, it seems, even if we only get it under the ingenious title of Cupid-and-Psychology.

LVII.
MEDICAL SCIENCE FOR WOMEN.

In reading, the other day, a speech on the Medical Education of Women, it struck me that the most important reason for this education was one which the speaker had not mentioned,—the fact that the medical profession stands for science; and that women peculiarly need science, since their natural bent is supposed to be a little the other way. The other professions represent tradition very generally: the lawyer must be bound by precedents; the clergyman generally admits that he must go back to his texts. But the physician claims, at least, to be a man of science, and stands for that before the world. Hence the sacredness with which his position has always been surrounded. The Florida Indians, according to the early voyagers, not only took the physician's medicine, but they took the physician himself internally, after his death. All other men were buried; but the body of the physician was burned, and his ashes mixed with water, by way of a permanent prescription.

At any rate, the physician himself popularly stands for science; and, in this point of view, his position is very noble. I have known physicians whose professed materialism was more elevated than most of what the world calls religion. To trace that wondrous power called life, which takes these particles of matter, and makes them think with thought, or glow with passion, or put forth an activity so intense as to be the parent of new life from generation to generation,—this study is something sublime. He who reverently ponders on this may call himself theist or atheist, he is yet worthy to be revered: if he can teach us, he blesses us. "I touch heaven," said Novalis, "when I lay my hand on a human body;" and the popularity among physicians of that fine engraving of Vesalius standing ready for his first dissection, shows that they take a higher view of their vocation than the world sometimes admits.

It seems to me peculiarly important that women should have a share in these studies. They often have time enough. It takes more time for a woman to make herself charming than to make herself learned, Sydney Smith says; and he thinks it a pity that she should often hang up her brains on the wall in poor pictures, or waft them into the air in poor music, when they might be better employed. Yet a great physician, Dr. Currie, says in his letters that he always preferred to have an ignorant patient bring his wife with him, because he could always get more careful observation and quicker suggestions from the woman. This point lies directly in the line of medical education.

The study lies also directly in their path as prospective wives and mothers, and this alone would furnish a sufficient reason for it. A woman of superior gifts, who had studied medicine, but never adopted it as a profession, told me that the mere domestic use of her knowledge had more than repaid her for all the trouble it had cost. For a man who should thus abandon the pursuit, it would be of comparatively little service, apart from the general training; but for a woman, if she fulfills the commoner duties of a woman's life, this early knowledge will always be a source of direct strength. This applies in a degree to surgery also; and I have always wondered, in view of the old proverb that a surgeon should have "a lion's heart and a lady's hand," why our professors do not oftener aim at developing this heart, if need be, in those who have the hand without training.

LVIII.
SEWING IN SCHOOLS.

Mr. N. T. Allen, of West Newton, Mass., who has had much experience and success as a teacher of both sexes, has been visiting the German public schools. He has lately given an interesting report of his observations to the Middlesex County Teachers' Association. The reporter says (the Italics being my own),—

"Mr. Allen paid particular attention to the Dorf Schule of the cities, and the Bürger Schule of the country, both being of the lower grades; and contended that the educational system of Germany was far from being perfect, and was inferior in certain respects to that adopted in some of our own States, and carried into successful operation in several towns and communities. It was compulsory and autocratic, in that parents were not allowed any choice in the education of their children; *it was unjust toward girls, in establishing and perpetuating the idea of their great mental inferiority to the boys*; it was undemocratic, in having different schools for different castes and classes of society; and it was extremely sectarian and bigoted in the religious dogmatic instruction prescribed and forced upon all."

It is well known that in the German schools a certain number of hours are given by the girls to sewing, and that their course of study, as compared with that of the boys, is narrowed to make room for this. It is for this reason that I, for one, dread to see sewing brought into our public schools. So strong is still the disposition in many minds to put off girls with less schooling than boys, that it seems unsafe to provide so good an excuse for this inequality.

The whole theory of industrial schools is liable to a similar danger,—that of introducing class distinctions into our education. It tends toward that other evil of the German system, described by Mr. Allen, "having different schools for different castes in society." I hold to the old theory of providing all boys and girls, whatever their parentage or probable pursuit, with a good basis of common-school education, and then trusting the intellectual faculties, thus sharpened, to help them in the struggle for life. Just as it was found in the army that a well-educated young man who had never handled a musket soon overtook and passed a comrade of inferior brains who had been in the militia from boyhood, so is it found to be with those whose minds have been well taught in our public schools. But whether this criticism holds, or not, against industrial schools, as such, it certainly holds when we further make an industrial discrimination against all girls. This we do, if we take an hour of their time for sewing, when the boys give that hour to study.

But it will be said, Ought not girls to be taught to sew? Undoubtedly. All boys ought to be taught the use of hammer and plane and screw-driver, and, for that matter, plain sewing also. Girls need sewing no doubt; and they should be taught it at home, or at school, or wherever they can find a teacher. But, for all this, to assign to sewing any thing like the same relative importance that belonged to it a hundred years ago, or even twenty years ago, is to overlook the changed conditions of modern society. Let us consider this a moment.

The Old-World theory was that all imaginable hard work was to be done by human hands. But the New-World theory is—for it is a New World wherever the theory is recognized—that all this work should be done, as far as possible, by human brains. Napoleon defined it as his ultimate intention for the French people, "to convert all trades into arts," the head doing the work of the hands. This applies to woman's work as much as any other. The epoch of private spinning and weaving was an epoch of barbarism; the vast mills of Lowell and Fall River now do that toil. The sewing-machine does a day's work in an hour. But all this machinery came out of somebody's brain, and is adapted to a race of women with brains. The treasurer of half a dozen manufacturing corporations told me last week, that, though the mills were filled with French and Irish, the superiority of American "help" was just as manifest as ever, and the manufacturers would gladly keep them if they could: they could almost always tend more looms, for instance. Those who have tried to teach the use of the sewing-machine to the Southern negroes or poor whites know how hard it is. A sewing-machine is a step in civilization: its presence in a house, like that of a piano, proves a certain stage of advancement. Its course runs parallel with that of the common-school; and an agent for this machine, like those who sell improved agricultural implements, would instinctively avoid those regions where there are no schoolhouses.

I do not undervalue the use of the hands, or the need of physical training for both boys and girls. But, after all, the hands must be kept subordinate to the head. If industrial training is to be the first thing, then every Irish parent who takes his ten-year-old girl from school, and sends her to the factory, is in the path of virtue. If, on the other hand, it be found that some time can be advantageously taken from books, and given to some handiwork, without loss of intellectual progress, that is a different thing. That is only an intellectual eight-hour bill or five-hour bill; and, for one, I should gladly favor that. But let it be done as securing the best education for all; not as a class-education, or as merely utilitarian: and let it be done as rigidly for boys as for girls. Let us not set out with the theory that a boy may avail himself of all the divisions of labor in modern society, but that every girl must still spin her own cloth, and sew her own seam.

LIX.
CASH PREMIUMS FOR STUDY.

On looking over the Harvard College catalogue, I am struck with the great pecuniary inducements which are held out to tempt young gentlemen to study. There are, to begin with, one hundred and seventeen "scholarships;" yielding incomes ranging from $40 to $350 annually, but averaging $225. The total income of these is $19,635. Then there are "loan" and "beneficiary" funds, amounting to $4,700 annually, and given or lent in sums from $25 to $75. Then there are "monitorships," yielding $700 per annum; and various money prizes, amounting to some $1,200. The whole amount that is or may be paid in cash to undergraduates every year is more than $25,000, which may perhaps reach a hundred and fifty young men. No wonder that the catalogue asserts that "The experience of the past warrants the statement that good scholars of high character, but slender means, are seldom or never obliged to leave college for want of money."

Probably one-sixth of the eight hundred undergraduates of Harvard College receive direct pecuniary aid in studying there; and, as scholarship is an essential in securing most of this pecuniary aid, it is probable that half the high scholars in every class are thus directly helped. Observe that this is in addition to the general value of the college endowments to all students, over and above what they pay for tuition,—an amount lately estimated by the academical authorities at one thousand dollars, at least, for every graduate. Apart from all this, I was told many years ago, by that very acute observer, the late President James Walker of Harvard University, that in his opinion one-quarter of the undergraduates were maintained in college through the personal self-denial and sacrifices of mothers and sisters.

But what a tremendous protective tariff, what an irresistible "discriminating duty," is this! While boys are thus bribed largely, year by year, to come to Cambridge, and study,—so that the influence of all this promise of pecuniary aid is felt through every academy and high school in the land,—we find, on the other hand, that every girl who wishes to pursue similar studies is expected to pay at the full market rates for all she gets, and even then cannot enter Harvard College. In some of our normal schools her board may be paid, I believe, on condition that she becomes a teacher; but I know of no place where she herself is paid, as young men are paid, merely to come and study. Ex-Gov. Bullock founded one scholarship at Amherst, of which the income is to be given by preference to a woman—when a woman is admitted! But unfortunately that time has not come. And yet those who sit by the banks of this golden stream, and monopolize all its benefits, have a tone of sublime contempt for those who are not permitted to approach it, and never can quite forgive the impecunious condition of these outcasts! "Your scholarship is not to be compared to ours," they say to women. "Certainly not," the women may fairly reply: "we were never paid salaries that we might become scholars."

The thing that perpetually neutralizes all claims of chivalry, all professions of justice, all talk of fairness, as between the sexes, is this class of facts. Woman is systematically excluded from training, and then told she must not compete; if admitted to compete, she is so weighted by artificial disadvantages, that it is hard for her to win. If her brain is inferior, she should be helped; if her natural obstacles are greater, all other hinderances should be the more generously swept away. Give girls a chance at a high school, they use it, and they there equal boys in scholarship; in our academies, in our normal schools, there is no deficiency on their part. Even in our colleges they ask, as yet, only admittance, not cash premiums. Only admit them, and see if they do not hold their own unpaid, with the young men to whom you pay, collectively, twenty-five thousand dollars a year to stay there. Only a seat in a recitation-room, to be paid for at the full price,—is this so very much for a young girl to ask? Do be at least as generous as that school committee in a Massachusetts town which shall be nameless, who said seriously in their report, speaking of a certain appointment, "As this place offers neither honor nor profit, we do not see why it should not be filled by a woman"!

LX.
MENTAL HORTICULTURE.

There was once a public meeting held, at the request of some excellent ladies, to consider the question whether it might be possible for roses and lilies to grow together in the same garden. Many of the ladies were quite used to gardening, and had opinions of their own; but, as it was not proper for them to open their lips before people, they of course could not testify. So several respectable gentlemen—clergymen and professors—were invited to tell them all about it. Some of these gentlemen had seen a rose, and some had seen a lily, but it turned out that very few of them had ever happened to see a garden. Still, as they were learned men, they could give very valuable suggestions. One of them explained, that, as roses and lilies assimilated very different juices from the soil, they could not possibly grow in the same soil. Another pointed out, that, as they needed different proportions of sun and of air, they should have very different exposures, and therefore must be kept apart. Another, more daring, suggested, that, as God had put the two species into the same world, it was quite possible that they might grow in the same enclosure for a time, perhaps for about fourteen years, but that, if they were left longer together, they would certainly blight and destroy each other. All this seemed very conclusive; and the meeting was about to vote that roses and lilies should never be allowed to exist in the same garden, unless with a brick wall twenty feet high between.

But it so happened that a sensible gardener from a distant State was present, and got up to say a word before the debate closed. "Bless your souls, my good people, what are you talking about?" said he. "Roses and lilies are already growing together by the thousand, all over the country, and you may as well close your discussion." Upon which the meeting broke up in some confusion: the brick wall was never built; but the clergyman went back to his study, the professor to his lecture-room, the physician to his patients, and all remained in the conviction that the gardener was a good sort of man, but strangely ignorant of scientific horticulture.

"Which things are an allegory." The writer has been reading the report, in the Boston Daily Advertiser, of a recent debate on female education.

I suppose that those born and bred in New England can never quite abandon the feeling that this region should still lead the nation, as it once led, in all educational matters. For one, I cannot help a slight sense of mortification, when, in an assemblage of Boston professors, undertaking to discuss a simple practical matter, everybody begins in the clouds, ignoring the facts before everybody's eyes, and discussing as a question of theory only, what has long since become a matter of common practice. The mortification is not diminished when the common-sense has to be at last imported from beyond the borders of New England, in the shape of a college president from Central New York. To him alone it seems to have occurred to remind these dwellers in the clouds that what they persisted in treating as theory had been a matter of daily experience in half the large towns in New England for the last quarter of a century.

What is the question at issue? Simply this: New England is full of normal schools, high schools, and endowed academies. In the majority of these, pupils of both sexes, from fourteen to twenty-five or thereabouts, study together and recite together, living either at home or in boarding-houses, or in academic dormitories, as the case may be. This has gone on for many years, without cavil or scandal. As a general rule, teachers have testified that they prefer to teach these mixed schools; at any rate, the fact is certain, that the sexes, once united in schools of this grade, are very seldom separated again; while we often hear of the separate schools as being abandoned, and the sexes brought together. Certainly the experiment of joint education has been very extensively tried in all parts of New England; indeed, for schools of this kind, in most regions, the association of the sexes is the rule, their separation the exception. Now, the only remaining question is: This being the case, will it make any essential difference if you widen the course of instruction a little, and call the institution a college?

This is really the only problem left to be solved; and yet on this question, thus limited, not a speaker at the above—except President White of Cornell University—had apparently a word to say. Every other speaker appeared to approach the general theme in as profound and blissful an ignorance as if he had lived all his life in Turkey or in France, or in some other country where no young man had ever recited algebra in the same room with a young woman since the world began.

EMPLOYMENT.

"The non-combatant population is sure to fare ill during the ages of combat. But these defects, too, are cured or lessened; women have now marvellous ways of winning their way in the world; and mind without muscle has far greater force than muscle without mind."—Bagehot's *Physics and Politics*, c. ii., § 3.

LXI.
"SEXUAL DIFFERENCE OF EMPLOYMENT."

I am at a loss to understand an assertion made by Rev. Dr. Hedge, at an educational meeting in Boston, that "the course of civilization hitherto has tended to develop and confirm sexual difference of employment." He adds, according to the report in the Daily Advertiser, that, "the more civilized the country, the more the vocations of men and women divide: the more savage the nation, the more they blend and coincide."

With due respect for Dr. Hedge on many grounds, and especially as having been the first man to demand publicly in presence of the Harvard alumni the admission of women to the university, I must yet express great surprise at his taking what seems to me so utterly untenable a position. To me it seems, on the contrary, that it is the savage period which is remarkable for the industrial separation of the sexes; and that every epoch of advancing civilization—as the present—blends them more and more. The fact would have seemed to me so plain as hardly to need more than simply to state it, but for the authority of Dr. Hedge upon the other side.

As we trace society back to savage life, what are the prevailing employments of the male sex? More and more exclusively, war and the chase. From these two vocations, monopolizing literally the whole active life of the savage man, the savage woman is almost absolutely excluded. Precisely at the point where the man's sphere leaves off, in each of these pursuits, the woman's sphere begins. Among American Indians, the man takes the captive, the woman tortures him. The man kills the deer, carries it till within sight of his own village, and then throws it down, that the squaw may go out and drag it in. Much that seems cruel and selfish in Indian life is the result, as Mrs. Jameson long since pointed out, of this complete separation of functions. The reason why the Indian woman carries the lodgepoles and the provisions on the march is that the man's limbs may be left free and agile for the far severer labors of war and of the chase, from which she is excluded. The reason why she finally brings the deer to the camp is because he has had the more exhausting labor of hunting and killing it.

Contrast now this absolute "sexual difference of employment" with the greater and greater blending of civilized society,—a blending, observe, which proceeds from both sides, and not from woman only. It is hard to say which is more remarkable, within the last half-century,—the way in which women have encroached on men's work, or the way in which men have encroached on women's.

In many mechanical and commercial pursuits,—as printing and bookkeeping,—once almost monopolized by men, you now find a very large number of women. In some pursuits, as in education, the women have come to outnumber the men enormously, at least in America; in others, as telegraphy, they seem likely to do the same. We constantly hear of new channels opening. A friend of mine, the other day, just before addressing an audience on woman suffrage, stepped into a barber's shop, and to his great amazement was shaved by a woman. On inquiry, he learned for the first time, that a good many of that sex, mostly Germans, pursued this occupation in New York and elsewhere. Thus do the vocations of men and women now "blend and coincide." On the other hand, the leading dressmaker of the world is a man; our bonnetshops are largely conducted by men; the eminent hotel cooks, whose salaries exceed any paid by Harvard University, are men; and the lady who goes to rest in a sleeping-car on our railroads has her pillow smoothed and her curtains drawn, not by a chambermaid, but by a chamberman.

These are the facts which seem to me, I must say, quite fatal to Dr. Hedge's theory. And there is one thing worth noticing in the very different criticisms passed on men and on women as to these invasions of each other's province. If you call attention to the way in which men are everywhere taking part in women's work, people say approvingly, "To be sure! greater energy, greater skill! they do even women's work better than women themselves can." But if you point out, that, on the other hand, women are also doing men's work, and in some cases—as in literature and lecturing—are actually obtaining higher prices than most men can obtain, the same people shake their heads disapprovingly, and say, "Unsexed; out of their sphere!" Now, if we lived in an age of chivalrous protection of women, it would be a different thing; but, as we live in an age of political economy, there is no reason why men alone should have the benefit of its laws. If practical life is to be regarded as a game of puss-in-the-corner, I should recommend to each ejected puss to make for the best corner she finds open, without much deference to the theories of the sages.

LXII.
THE USE OF ONE'S FEET.

Is it better to stand on one's own feet, or to depend on those of other people? We need clear views on that matter, certainly; and there is not much doubt which theory will ultimately prevail.

For one, I believe the whole theory of a leisure-class, whether for man or woman, to be a snare and a delusion. It seems to me that there is one great drawback that a young American may encounter,—namely, the possession of an independent property; and that there is one great piece of good fortune,—to be thrown on one's self for support. Of all influences for development or usefulness, I know of none so great as "the wholesome stimulus of pecuniary necessity." Of all forms of social organization, that seems to me the most favorable which opens to all most freely the opportunity of early education, and then calls upon each to exert himself for his own support.

To be sure, it is hardly possible to overrate the value of cultivated companionship and refined association. In other countries it may be worth while, for the sake of these, to be born to wealth: it is so hard to get them without wealth. But the happiest and best American households are apt to be found among such as Miss Alcott, for instance, habitually describes, where there is plenty of refinement and very little money; where perhaps there has been wealth in times past, but it has been lost just in time for the good of the children. All that money can bring—all books, all travel, all art—are not worth so much as the power to stand on one's own feet. It is an essential to the character, and it is certainly the greatest of delights. To have earned, for a single year, one's own support, gives one, in a manner, the freedom of the universe. Till that is done, we are children: after that we are mature human beings.

In England, where the whole social atmosphere is so different, there are many instances of much service done to art and philanthropy by persons born to leisure. And yet, even in England, if the admissions of English people may be trusted, these instances are bought by a frightful disproportion of wasted lives; and the best work is, after all, done by those who have learned to stand on their own feet. This last fact is certainly true of France, Germany, and America. So far as my own observation goes, for one American born to leisure who makes a good use of it, there are a dozen who lead empty or vicious lives. And even that exceptional one, with all his advantages, is often distanced in the race by the men who have early had to stand on their own feet. The man of leisure is usually so limited, either by the absence of stimulus or by the tiresome narrowness of a petty circle, or by missing the wholesome attrition of other minds, that he dwindles and grows feeble. If such a man attains by the aid of wealth what the man of the next inferior grade attains without it, we are all glad, and say it is "an honorable instance." Not that the rich are worse than other men. It is no calamity to earn wealth, or even to inherit it after we have learned the lesson of self-reliance. It is the children of wealth who are to be pitied.

Now, all women who are born outside of actual poverty in America are as badly off as if they had been born to wealth. They are systematically discouraged from the delightful tonic of self-support. But when it is said that they never even feel the desire to support themselves, I must dissent. For twenty years I have been encountering young women who so longed for the sense of an independent position that even the happiest paternal home could not satisfy them unless it gave them so much to do that they might honestly feel that they earned their living. Otherwise the most luxurious arm-chairs in their own houses would not satisfy them, they so longed to learn the use of their own feet. I have known girls to rejoice in their father's loss of property, because it would release them to enjoy the happiness of self-reliance; and, for one, had I the good fortune to have a dozen daughters, I should wish them all to be of this way of thinking. Any other theory would give us a world of mere amateurs and dilettantes, and very little work would be done. We are getting over the theory that it is undignified for a man to stand upon his own feet; and we shall one day get over it in regard to women.

LXIII.
MISS INGELOW'S PROBLEM.

In a certain New England town I lived opposite the house of a thriving mechanic. His wife, a young and pretty woman, soon attracted the attention of my household by the grace and vivacity of her bearing, and the peculiar tastefulness of her own and her little boy's costume. On further acquaintance, we found that she did every atom of her housework, washing and all; that she cut and made every garment for herself and her child; and that, finding her energies still unsatisfied, she took in sewing-work from a tailor's shop, and thus earned most of the money for their wardrobe. It may be well to add, to complete this story of New England social life, that her husband was one of the very earliest volunteers for the war of the Rebellion; that he went in captain, came out brigadier-general, and now holds an important government office.

There is nothing isolated or unexampled about this instance. My pretty and ladylike neighbor was only energetic, ready, capable, and ambitious, or, to sum it all up in the New England vernacular, "smart." Whatever she saw in society or life that was desirable for herself or her husband or her child, that she aimed at, and generally obtained.

She "hadn't a lazy bone in her body;" and she never will have, though she may wear that body out prematurely by nervous tension. Wherever she goes, she will carry the same restless, tireless energy; and, should her husband ever go to Congress or to the Court of St. James, she will carry herself with perfect fearlessness and ease. And in all this she represents one great type of New England women.

When you ask of such a woman if she shrinks from work, it is as if you asked, Does a deer shrink from running, or a swallow from flying? She loves the work: indeed she loves it, in my opinion, far too much, and sets a dangerous example. All theories of the natural indolence of man—or woman—fall defeated before the New England temperament, traditions, training, climate; before that "whip of the sky," as a poet has sung, that urges us on. If, therefore, "household work is thought degrading,"—and Miss Ingelow asserts too hastily that "nowhere is this so much the case as in America,"—it certainly is not merely because it is work.

For myself, I doubt the fact, and demand the evidence. So far as the free States of the Union are concerned, it seems to me that household labor is thought less degrading than in England, and that the proportion of well-taught and ladylike women who contentedly do their own work is far greater in America, and keeps pace with the greater spread of average education. There is not a city in the land, I suppose,—certainly not a village,—where the housework in a large majority of the American-born families is not done by Americans; for the large majority are always mechanics and laborers, among whom, as a rule, the work is done by the wives and sisters and daughters. The wages of domestics are so much higher in America than in England,—being almost double,—that it is here a more serious expenditure to employ such aid.

I think, therefore, that we must be very cautious before we say that housework, as such, is held degrading in the free States. No doubt, American women feel, as their husbands and brothers feel, that all work should be done by machinery, as far as possible, and that the washing-machine and the carpet-sweeper are as legitimate as the patent reaper or mower. They would be foolish if they did not. They also feel, as American men feel, that, in this great assemblage of all nations, the place for the American is rather in posts of command than in the ranks. In our ships you find men of all nations in the forecastle, but Americans in the cabin. In the regular army it is the officers, commissioned or non-commissioned, who are Americans. Go as far west as you please, you are surprised to find that the railway officials, superintendents, conductors, baggage-masters, are not merely American-born but often New-England-born. The better average education tells. It is in the fitness of things that the under-work of household life also should be done by the under-class of foreign elements, and that it should be Americans who do the direction and guidance. Some such instinct as this is the explanation of much that Miss Ingelow takes for a contempt of household labor. An American woman does not despise such labor, properly speaking, any more than an American man despises mechanical labor. Both aim, if they can, to rise to occupations more lucrative and more intellectual.

It is not the labor, it is not even the household labor, to which objection is made. When you come to household labor for other people, done in a capacity recognized as menial,—ay, there's the rub! There is a widespread feeling that domestic service in other people's families is menial.

For one I have publicly remonstrated against the excess of this feeling, and think it is carried too far. Women will never compete equally with men, until they are willing, like men, to do any honest work without sense of degradation. This is one point where enfranchisement will help them. So long as a man bears in his hand the ballot, that symbol of substantial equality, his self-respect is not easily impaired by the humblest position. "A man's a man for a' that," he knows, before the law. But a woman, not having this, has only the usages of society to guide her; and, so long as society talks about "master" and "servant," I do not blame the American girl for refusing to accept such a position,—just as I do not blame, but applaud, the American man for refusing to wear livery. I only condemn them, in either case, when the alternative is starvation or sin. Then pride should yield.

But this is the conclusive proof that it is not the housework which is held degrading: the fact that there is no difficulty in securing any number of American girls in our large country hotels, where they associate with their employers as equals, and call no man master. The fact that the proprietors of such hotels invariably prefer American "help" to Irish, shows that the philosophy of the whole question lies in a different direction from that indicated by our good friend Miss Ingelow. The evil of which she speaks does not properly exist: the real difficulty lies in a different direction, and cannot be settled till we see farther into the social organization that is to come.

LXIV.
SELF-SUPPORT.

It is the English theory, that society needs a leisure class, not self-supporting, from whom public services and works of science and art may proceed. Even Darwin recognizes this theory. But how little is England doing for science and art, compared to Germany! and the German work of that kind is not done by a leisure class, but by poor men. I believe that the necessity of self-support, at least in the earlier years of life, is the best training for manhood; and it does not seem desirable that women should be wholly set free from it.

A clever writer, on the other hand, maintains in the New York Independent that women should never support themselves if it be possible honorably to avoid it. "Pecuniary dependence, degrading to men, is not only not undignified, but is the only thoroughly dignified condition, for women. In a renovated and millennial society all women will be supported by men, —will have no more to do with bringing in money than the lilies of the field." This statement is delightfully uncompromising, and it is a great thing to hear an extreme position so clearly and unequivocally put. Especially on a question so difficult as the labor and wages of women, it is particularly desirable to have each extreme worked out to its logical results.

It is certainly the normal condition of woman to be a wife and a mother. It is equally certain that this condition withdraws woman from the labor-market, during the prime of her life. The very years during which a man attains his highest skill, and earns his highest wages,—say, from twenty-five to forty,—are lost to woman, in this normal condition, so far as earning money is concerned. This is the main fact, as I judge, which keeps down the standard of both work and pay among women, as a class. If men, as a class, were thus heavily weighted, the result would be as clearly seen. Where one sex brings into the market the full vigor of its life, and the other has only crude labor, or occasional labor, or broken labor, to offer, the result cannot be doubtful. Yet this is precisely the state of the competition between man and woman.

I believe, therefore, with this writer, that woman was not intended to be the equal competitor of man in business pursuits—or, indeed, to be self-supporting at all—during her career of motherhood. It is generally recognized as a calamity, when she is obliged to support herself at that time. Most people believe with Miss Mitford that "women were not meant to earn the bread of a family," and that men are. But to earn the bread of a family is not self-support: it is much more than self-support. And when this writer takes a step beyond, and says, "I think the necessity of earning her own living is always a woman's misfortune," then she seems to theorize beyond good sense, and to confuse things very different. Self-support is one thing: supporting seven small children is quite another thing.

That which should never be left out of sight is the essential dignity of labor. Woman during the period of maternity is rightly excused from earning money; but it is because she is better occupied. She is not exempted in the character of lily of the field, but in the capacity of mother of a family. It is an important distinction. For labor in the lower sense, she substitutes what, in a higher and more sacred sense, we still call "labor." She is not supported because she is a woman, but because, in her capacity as woman, she happens to have home-duties. If she had no such duties, there seems no reason why she should be supported any more than if she were a man. To be a wife and mother is a vocation, and one which usually for a time precludes all others. Merely to be a woman is not a vocation; and, so long as one can make no better claim on the world than that, the world has a right to demand something more. The Irishwoman who locks her little children into her one room, that she may go out to earn their bread, seems to me in a position no falser than that of the over-worked father who breaks himself down with toil that his daughters may live like the lilies of the field.

LXV.
SELF-SUPPORTING WIVES.

For one, I have never been fascinated by the style of domestic paradise that English novels depict,—half a dozen unmarried daughters round the family hearth, all assiduously doing worsted-work and petting their papa. I believe a sufficiency of employment to be the only normal and healthy condition for a human being; and where there is not work enough to employ the full energies of all, at home, it seems as proper for young women as for young birds to leave the parental nest. If this additional work is done for money, very well. It is the conscious dignity of self-support that removes the traditional curse from labor, and woman has a right to claim her share in that dignified position.

Yet I cannot agree, on the other hand, with Celia Burleigh when she says that her "True Woman" should be self-supporting, even in marriage. Women's part of the family task—the care of home and children—is just as essential to building up the family fortunes as the very different toil of the out-door partner. For young married women to undertake any more direct aid to the family income is in most cases utterly undesirable, and is asking of themselves a great deal too much. And this is not because they are to be encouraged in indolence, but because they already, in a normal condition of things, have their hands full. As, on this point, I may differ from some of my readers, let me explain precisely what I mean.

As I write, there are at work, in another part of the house, two paper-hangers, a man and his wife, each forty-five or fifty years of age. Their children are grown up, and some of them married: they have a daughter at home, who is old enough to do the housework, and leave the mother free. There is no way of organizing the labors of this household better than this: the married pair toil together during the day, and go home together to their evening rest. A happier couple I never saw; it is a delight to see them cheerily at work together, cutting, pasting, hanging: their life seems like a prolonged industrial picnic; and, if I had the ill-luck to own as many palaces as an English duke, I should keep them permanently occupied in putting fresh papers on the walls.

But the merit of this employment for the woman is, that it interferes with no other duty. Were she a young mother with little children, and obliged by her paper-hanging to neglect them, or to leave them at a "day-nursery," or to overwork herself by combining too many cares, then the sight of her would be very sad. So sacred a thing does motherhood seem to me, so paramount and absorbing the duty of a mother to her child, that in a true state of society I think she should be utterly free from all other duties,—even, if possible, from the ordinary cares of housekeeping. If she has spare health and strength to do these other things as pleasures, very well; but she should be relieved from them as duties. And, as to the need of self-support, I can hardly conceive of an instance where it can be to the mother of young children any thing but a disaster. As we all know, this calamity often occurs; I have seen it among the factory-operatives at the North, and among the negro-women in the cotton-fields at the South: in both cases it is a tragedy, and the bodies and brains of mother and children alike suffer. That the mother should bear and tend and nurture, while the father supports and protects,—this is the true division.

Does this bear in any way upon suffrage? Not at all. The mother can inform herself upon public questions in the intervals of her cares, as the father among his; and the baby in the cradle is a perpetual appeal to her, as to him, that the institutions under which that baby dwells may be kept pure. One of the most devoted young mothers I ever knew—the younger sister of Margaret Fuller Ossoli—made it a rule, no matter how much her children absorbed her, to read books or newspapers for an hour every day; in order, she said, that their mother should be more than a mere source of physical nurture, and that her mind should be kept fresh and alive for them. But to demand in addition that such a mother should earn money for them, is to ask too much; and there is many a tombstone in New England, which, if it told the truth, would tell what comes of such an effort.

LXVI.
THE PROBLEM OF WAGES.

Talking, the other day, with one of the leading dressmakers of a New England town, I asked her why it was, that, when women suffered so much from scanty employments and low pay, there should yet be so few good dressmakers. "You are all overrun and worn out with work," I said, "all the year round; every lady in town complains that there are so few of you; and it is the same in every town where I ever lived." She answered, as such witnesses always answer, "Women do not engage in occupations, as men do, for a lifetime. They expect only to continue in them for a year or two, until they shall be married. I employ twelve girls, and not one of them expects to be a dressmaker for life. They work their ten hours a day, under my direction, and that is all."

Here lies the point of difference between the work of women and that of men, as a class: I mean, in their industrial pursuits, the work that earns money. Until we reach this point, or get a social philosophy that explains this, we are yet upon the surface only. The enfranchisement of woman will help us towards this, but will not, of itself, solve the problem of wages; because that depends on other than political considerations.

Why do the mass of men work? Not from taste, or for love of the work, but from conscious need. If they do not work, they and their families will starve. It is a necessity, and a permanent necessity. It will last all their lives, except in the case of a few who will "come into their property" by and by, like Mr. Toots—and their work is usually worth about as much as his. We see this every day in the sons of rich men. Their fathers may bring them up to work, yet the mere fact that they are to be relieved from this compulsion within a dozen years is apt to paralyze their active faculties. They study law or medicine, or dabble in "business;" but they only play at the practice of their pursuits, because there is no conscious necessity behind them. There are exceptions, but the exceptions are remarkable men.

Now, theorize as we may, the fact at present is, that what thus paralyzes the energies of a few young men brings the same paralysis to many young women. Those whose parents are wealthy do not learn any regular occupation at all. Those whose parents are poor are obliged by necessity to learn one: yet they do not learn it as men in general learn theirs, but only as rich young men do, as if it were something to be followed for a time only,—till they "come into their property." To the rich young man the property is a landed estate or some bank-stock. To the poor girl the prospective property is a husband. She expects to be married; and after that her money-making occupation is gone, and a new avocation—that of housekeeping and maternity—begins. It is no less arduous, no less honorable; but it is different. In it her previous special training goes for nothing; and the thought of this must diminish her interest in the previous special training. It is only a temporary thing, like the few years' labor of a rich young man. There are exceptions, but they are extraordinary.

One reason why women's work is not at present so well paid as that of men is because it is not ordinarily so well done, especially in the more difficult parts. All employers, male and female, tell you this; and one great reason why it is not so well done is because women have not, as men have, a spring of permanent necessity to urge them on. How shall we supply the spring? This is the question we need to answer. As yet I do not think we have reached it. It does not seem to me to be, like the suffrage question, one easily settled. The reader will find very important facts and testimonies bearing upon it in Virginia Penny's "Cyclopædia of Female Employments."[13]

13. Especially on pp. 110, 146, 235, 238, 243, 245, 247, 300, 318, 322, 367, 380.

I confess myself unable, even after a good many years of study, to solve it fully; but a few propositions, I think, are sure, and may be taken as axioms to begin with. The general wages of women will always depend greatly on the amount of skill acquired by the mass of them. The mass of women will always look forward to being married, and, when married, to being necessarily withdrawn from the labor-market. Those who look forward to this withdrawal will not, as a rule, concentrate themselves upon learning their vocation as if it were for life; and, at any rate, when they leave it, they will take their skill with them, and so lower the average skill of the whole.

The problem, therefore, is, how to equalize wages between a sex which works continually throughout life, driven by conscious necessity, and a sex which habitually works with temporary expectations, looking forward to a withdrawal from the labor-market in a few years, and which, when so withdrawn, carries its acquired skill with it, leaving only inexperience in its place. We all wish to solve the problem: every man would like to have his daughters as well paid for their labor as his sons. The ballot will help to elucidate it, no doubt, by putting woman's political protection, at least, into her own hands: but wholly to solve the problem will take the wisdom of several generations; nor will it be done, perhaps, until the greater problem of association *vs.* competition is also understood. It certainly never will be solved by slighting the marriage-relation, or by advocating either "free love" or celibacy for women or for men.

LXVII.
THOROUGH.

"The hopeless defect of women in all practical matters," said a shrewd merchant the other day, "is, that it is impossible to make them thorough." It was a shallow remark, and so I told him. Women are thorough in the things which they have accepted as their sphere,—in their housekeeping and their dress and their social observances. There is nothing more thorough on earth than the way housework is done in a genuine New England household. There is an exquisite thoroughness in the way a milliner's or a dressmaker's work is done,—a work such as clumsy man cannot rival, and can hardly estimate. No general plans his campaigns or marshals his armies better than some women of society manage the circles of which they are the centre. Day and night, winter and summer, at city or watering-place, year in and year out, such a woman keeps open house for her gay world. She has a perpetual series of guests who must be fed luxuriously, and amused profusely; she talks to them in four or five languages; at her entertainments, she notes who is present and who absent, as carefully as Napoleon watched his soldiers; her interchange of cards, alone, is a thing as complex as the army muster-rolls: thus she plans, organizes, conquers, and governs. People speak of her existence as that of a doll or a toy, when she is the most untiring of campaigners. Grant that her aim is, after all, unworthy, and that you pity the worn face which has to force so many smiles. No matter: the smiles are there, and so is the success. I often wish that the reformers would do their work as thoroughly as the women of society do theirs.

No, there is no constitutional want of thoroughness in women. The trouble is, that into the new work upon which they are just entering, they have not yet brought their thoroughness to bear. They suffer and are defrauded and are reproached, simply because they have not yet nerved themselves to do well the things which they have asserted their right to do. A distinguished woman, who earns perhaps the largest income ever honestly earned by any woman off the stage, told me the other day that she left all her business affairs to the management of others, and did not even know how to draw a check on a bank. What a melancholy self-exhibition was that of a clever American woman, the author of half a dozen successful books, refusing to look her own accounts in the face until they had got into such a tangle that not even her own referees could disentangle them to suit her! These things show, not that women are constitutionally wanting in thoroughness, but that it is hard to make them carry this quality into new fields.

I wish I could possibly convey to the young women who write for advice on literary projects something of the meaning of this word "thorough" as applied to literary work. Scarcely any of them seem to have a conception of it. Dash, cleverness, recklessness, impatience of revision or of patient investigation, these are the common traits. To a person of experience, no stupidity is so discouraging as a brilliancy that has no roots. It brings nothing to pass; whereas a slow stupidity, if it takes time enough, may conquer the world. Consider that for more than twenty years the path of literature has been quite as fully open for women as for men, in America,— the payment the same, the honor the same, the obstacles no greater. Collegiate education has until very lately been denied them, but how many men succeed as writers without that advantage! Yet how little, how very little, of really good literary work has yet been done by American women! Young girls appear one after another: each writes a single clever story or a single sweet poem, and then disappears forever. Look at Griswold's "Female Poets of America," and you are disposed to turn back to the title-page, and see if these utterly forgotten names do not really represent the "female poets" of some other nation. They are forgotten, as most of the more numerous "female prose writers" are forgotten, because they had no root. Nobody doubts that women have cleverness enough, and enough of power of expression. If you could open the mails, and take out the women's letters, as somebody says, they would prove far more graphic and entertaining than those of the men. They would be written, too, in what Macaulay calls—speaking of Madame d'Arblay's early style—"true woman's English, clear, natural, and lively." What they need, in order to convert this epistolary brilliancy into literature, is to be thorough.

You cannot separate woman's rights and her responsibilities. In all ages of the world she has had a certain limited work to do, and has done that well. All that is needed, when new spheres are open, is that she should carry the same fidelity into those. If she will work as hard to shape the children of her brain as to rear her bodily offspring, will do intellectual work as well as she does housework, and will meet her moral responsibilities as she meets her social engagements, then opposition will soon disappear. The habit of thoroughness is the key to all high success. Whatever is worth doing is worth doing well. Only those who are faithful in a few things will rightfully be made rulers over many.

LXVIII.
LITERARY ASPIRANTS.

The brilliant Lady Ashburton used to say of herself that she had never written a book, and knew nobody whose book she would like to have written. This does not seem to be the ordinary state of mind among those who write letters of inquiry to authors. If I may judge from these letters, the yearning for a literary career is just now greater among women than among men. Perhaps it is because of some literary successes lately achieved by women. Perhaps it is because they have fewer outlets for their energies. Perhaps they find more obstacles in literature than young men find, and have, therefore, more need to write letters of inquiry about it. It is certain that they write such letters quite often; and ask questions that test severely the supposed omniscience of the author's brain,—questions bearing on logic, rhetoric, grammar, and orthography; how to find a publisher, and how to obtain a well-disciplined mind.

These letters may sometimes be too long or come too often for convenience, nor is the consoling postage-stamp always remembered. But they are of great value as giving real glimpses of American social life, and of the present tendencies of American women. They sometimes reveal such intellectual ardor and imagination, such modesty, and such patience under difficulties, as to do good to the reader, whatever they may do to the writer. They certainly suggest a few thoughts, which may as well be expressed, once for all, in print.

Behind almost all these letters there lies a laudable desire to achieve success. "Would you have the goodness to tell us how success can be obtained?" How can this be answered, my dear young lady, when you leave it to the reader to guess what your definition of success may be? For instance, here is Mr. Mansfield Tracy Walworth, who was murdered the other day in New York. He was at once mentioned in the newspapers as a "celebrated author." Never in my life having heard of him, I looked in Hart's "Manual of American Literature," and there found that Mr. Walworth's novel of "Warwick" had a sale of seventy-five thousand copies, and his "Delaplaine" of forty-five thousand. Is it a success to have secured a sale like that for your books, and then to die, and have your brother penmen ask, "Who was he?" Yet, certainly, a sale of seventy-five thousand copies is not to be despised; and I fear I know many youths and maidens who would willingly write novels much poorer than "Warwick" for the sake of a circulation like that. I do not think that Hawthorne, however, would have accepted these conditions; and he certainly did not have this style of success.

Nor do I think he had any right to expect it. He had made his choice, and had reason to be satisfied. The very first essential for literary success is to decide what success means. If a young girl pines after the success of Marion Harland and Mrs. Southworth, let her seek it. It is possible that she may obtain it, or surpass it; and, though she might do better, she might do far worse. It is, at any rate, a laudable aim to be popular: popularity may be a very creditable thing, unless you pay too high a price for it. It is a pleasant thing, and has many contingent advantages,—balanced by this great danger, that one is apt to mistake it for success.

"Learning hath made the most," said old Fuller, "by those books on which the booksellers have lost." If this be true of learning, it is quite as true of genius and originality. A book may be immediately popular and also immortal, but the chances are the other way. It is more often the case, that a great writer gradually creates the taste by which he is enjoyed. Wordsworth in the last generation and Emerson in the present have been striking instances of this; and authors of far less fame have yet the same choice which they had. You can take the standard which the book-market offers, and train yourself for that. This will, in the present age, be sure to educate certain qualities in you,—directness, vividness, animation, dash,—even if it leaves other qualities untrained. Or you can make a standard of your own, and aim at that, taking your chance of seeing the public agree with you. Very likely you may fail; perhaps you may be wrong in your fancy, after all, and the public may be right: if you fail, you may find it hard to bear; but, on the other hand, you may have the inward "glory and joy" which nothing but fidelity to an ideal standard can give. All this applies to all forms of work, but it applies conspicuously to literature.

Instead, therefore, of offering to young writers the usual comforting assurance, that, if they produce any thing of real merit, it will be sure to succeed, I should caution them first to make their own definition of success, and then act accordingly. Hawthorne succeeded in his way, and Mr. M. T. Walworth in his way; and each of these would have been very unreasonable if he had expected to succeed in both ways. There is always an opening for careful and conscientious literary work; and, by such work, many persons obtain a modest support. There are also some great prizes to be won; but these are commonly, though not always, won by work of a more temporary and sensational kind. Make your choice; and, when you have got precisely what you asked for, do not complain because you have missed what you would not take.

LXIX.
"THE CAREER OF LETTERS."

A young girl of some talent once told me that she had devoted herself to "the career of letters." I found, on inquiry, that she had obtained a situation as writer of "society" gossip for a New York newspaper. I can hardly imagine any life that leads more directly away from any really literary career, or any life about which it is harder to give counsel. The work of a newspaper-correspondent, especially in the "society" direction, is so full of trials and temptations, for one of either sex, in our dear, inquisitive, gossiping America, that one cannot help watching with especial solicitude all women who enter it. Their special gifts as women are a source of danger: they are keener of observation from the very fact of their sex, more active in curiosity, more skilful in achieving their ends; in a world of gossip they are the queens, and men but their subjects, hence their greater danger.

In Newport, New York, Washington, it is the same thing. The unbounded appetite for private information about public or semi-public people creates its own purveyors; and these, again, learn to believe with unflinching heartiness in the work they do. I have rarely encountered a successful correspondent of this description who had not become thoroughly convinced that the highest desire of every human being is to see his name in print, no matter how. Unhappily there is a great deal to encourage this belief: I have known men to express great indignation at an unexpected newspaper-puff, and then to send ten dollars privately to the author. This is just the calamity of the profession, that it brings one in contact with this class of social hypocrites; and the "personal" correspondent gradually loses faith that there is any other class to be found. Then there is the perilous temptation to pay off grudges in this way, to revenge slights, by the use of a power with which few people are safely to be trusted. In many cases, such a correspondent is simply a child playing with poisoned arrows: he poisons others; and it is no satisfaction to know that in time he will also poison himself, and paralyze his own power for mischief.

There lies before me a letter written some years ago to a young lady anxious to enter on this particular "career of letters,"—a letter from an experienced New York journalist. He has employed, he says, hundreds of lady correspondents, for little or no compensation; and one of his few successful writers he thus describes: "She succeeds by pushing her way into society, and extracting information from fashionable people and officials and their wives.... She flatters the vain, and overawes the weak, and gets by sheer impudence what other writers cannot.... I would not wish you to be like her, or reduced to the necessity of doing what she does, for any success journalism can possibly give." And who can help echoing this opinion? If this is one of the successful laborers, where shall we place the unsuccessful; or, rather, is success, or failure, the greater honor?

Personal journalism has a prominence in this country with which nothing in any other country can be compared. What is called publicity in England or France means the most peaceful seclusion, compared with the glare of notoriety which an enterprising correspondent can flash out at any time—as if by opening the bull's-eye of a dark lantern—upon the quietest of his contemporaries. It is essentially an American institution, and not one of those in which we have reason to feel most pride. It is to be observed, however, that foreigners, if in office, take to it very readily; and it is said that no people cultivate the reporters at Washington more assiduously than the diplomatic corps, who like to send home the personal notices of themselves, in order to prove to their governments that they are highly esteemed in the land to which they are appointed. But, however it may be with them, it is certain that many people still like to keep their public and private lives apart, and shrink from even the inevitable eminence of fame. One of the very most popular of American authors has said that he never, to this day, has overcome a slight feeling of repugnance on seeing his own name in print.

LXX.
TALKING AND TAKING.

Every time a woman does any thing original or remarkable,—inventing a rat-trap, let us say, or carving thirty-six heads on a walnut-shell,—all observers shout applause. "There's a woman for you, indeed! Instead of talking about her rights, she takes them. That's the way to do it. What a lesson to these declaimers upon the platform!"

It does not seem to occur to these wise people that the right to talk is itself one of the chief rights in America, and the way to reach all the others. To talk, is to make a beginning, at any rate. To catch people with your ideas, is more than to contrive a rat-trap; and Isotta Nogarola, carving thirty-six empty heads, was not working in so practical a fashion as Mary Livermore when she instructs thirty-six hundred full ones.

It shows the good sense of the woman suffrage agitators, that they have decided to begin with talk. In the first place, talking is the most lucrative of all professions in America; and therefore it is the duty of American women to secure their share of it. Mrs. Frances Anne Kemble used to say that she read Shakspeare in public "for her bread;" and when, after melting all hearts by a course of farewell readings, she decided to begin reading again, she said she was doing it "for her butter." So long as women are often obliged to support themselves and their children, and perhaps their husbands, by their own labor, they have no right to work cheaply, unless driven to it. Anna Dickinson has no right to make fifteen dollars a week by sewing, if, by stepping out of the ranks of needle-women into the ranks of the talkers, she can make a hundred dollars a day. Theorize as we may, the fact is, that there is no kind of work in America which brings such sure profits as public speaking. If women are unfitted for it, or if they "know the value of peace and quietness," as the hand-organ-man says, and can afford to hold their tongues, let them do so. But if they have tongues, and like to use them, they certainly ought to make some money by the performance.

This is the utilitarian view. And when we bring in higher objects, it is plain that the way to get any thing in America is to talk about it. Silence is golden, no doubt, and like other gold remains in the bank-vaults, and does not just now circulate very freely as currency. Even literature in America is utterly second to oratory as a means of immediate influence. Of all sway, that of the orator is the most potent and most perishable; and the student and the artist are apt to hold themselves aloof from it, for this reason. But it is the one means in America to accomplish immediate results, and women who would take their rights must take them through talking. It is the appointed way.

Under a good old-fashioned monarchy, if a woman wished to secure any thing for her sex, she must cajole a court, or become the mistress of a monarch. That epoch ended with the French Revolution. When Bonaparte wished to silence Madame de Staël, he said, "What does that woman want? Does she want the money the government owes to her father?" When Madame de Staël heard of it, she said, "The question is not what I want, but what I think." Henceforth women, like men, are to say what they think. For all that flattery and seduction and sin, we have substituted the simple weapon of talk. If women wish education, they must talk; if better laws, they must talk. The one chief argument against woman suffrage, with men, is that so few women even talk about it.

As long as talk can effect any thing, it is the duty of women to talk; and in America, where it effects every thing, they should talk all the time. When they have obtained, as a class, absolute equality of rights with men, their talk on this subject may be silent, and they may accept, if they please, that naughty masculine definition of a happy marriage,—the union of a deaf man with a dumb woman.

LXXI.
HOW TO SPEAK IN PUBLIC.

There are other things that women wish to do, it seems, beside studying and voting. There are a good many—if I may judge from letters that occasionally come to me—who are taking, or wish to take, their first lessons in public speaking. Not necessarily very much in public, or before mixed audiences, but perhaps merely to say to a room-full of ladies, or before the committee of a Christian Union, what they desire to say. "How shall I make myself heard? How shall I learn to express myself? How shall I keep my head clear? Is there any school for debate?" And so on. My dear young lady, it does not take much wisdom, but only a little experience, to answer some of these questions. So I am not afraid to try.

The best school for debate is debating. So far as mere confidence and comfort are concerned, the great thing is to gain the habit of speech, even if one speaks badly. And the practice of an ordinary debating society has also this advantage, that it teaches you to talk sense (lest you be laughed at), to speak with some animation (lest your hearers go to sleep), to think out some good arguments (because you are trying to convince somebody), and to guard against weak reasoning or unfounded assertion (lest your opponent trip you up). Speaking in a debating society thus gives you the same advantage that a lawyer derives from the presence of an opposing counsel: you learn to guard yourself at all points. It is the absence of this check which is the great intellectual disadvantage of the pulpit. When a lawyer says a foolish thing in an argument, he is pretty sure to find it out; but a clergyman may go on repeating his foolish thing for fifty years without finding it out, for want of an opponent.

For the art of making your voice heard, I must refer you to an elocutionist. Yet one thing at least you might acquire for yourself,—a thing that lies at the foundation of all good speaking,—the complete and thorough enunciation of every syllable. So great is the delight, to my ear at least, of a perfectly distinct and clear-cut utterance, that I fear I should rather listen for an hour to the merest nonsense, so uttered, than to the very wisdom of angels if given in a confused or nasal or slovenly way. If you wish to know what I mean by a clear and satisfactory utterance, go to the next woman suffrage convention, and hear Miss Eastman.

As to your employment of language, the great aim is to be simple, and, in a measure, conversational, and then let eloquence come of itself. If most people talked as well in public as in private, public meetings would be more interesting. To acquire a conversational tone, there is good sense in Edward Hale's suggestion, that every person who is called on to speak,—let us say, at a public dinner,—instead of standing up and talking about his surprise at being called on, should simply make his last remark to his neighbor at the table the starting-point for what he says to the whole company. He will thus make sure of a perfectly natural key, to begin with; and can go on from this quiet "As I was just saying to Mr. Smith," to discuss the gravest question of Church or State. It breaks the ice for him, like the remark upon the weather by which we open our interview with the person whom we have longed for years to meet. Beginning in this way at the level of the earth's surface, we can join hands and rise to the clouds. Begin in the clouds,—as some of my most esteemed friends are wont to do,—and you have to sit down before reaching the earth.

And, to come last to what is first in importance, I am taking it for granted that you have something to say, and a strong desire to say it. Perhaps you can say it better for writing it out in full beforehand. But, whether you do this or not, remember that the more simple and consecutive your thought, the easier it will be both to keep it in mind and to utter it. The more orderly your plan, the less likely you will be to "get bewildered," or to "lose the thread." Think it out so clearly that the successive parts lead to one another, and then there will be little strain upon your memory. For each point you make, provide at least one good argument and one good illustration, and you can, after a little practice, safely leave the rest to the suggestion of the moment. But so much as this you must have, to be secure. Methods of preparation of course vary extremely; yet I suppose the secret of the composure of an experienced speaker to lie usually in this, that he has made sure beforehand of a sufficient number of good points to carry him through, even if nothing good should occur to him on the spot. Thus wise people, in going on a fishing-excursion, take with them not merely their fishing-tackle, but a few fish; and then, if they are not sure of their luck, they will be sure of their chowder.

These are some of the simple hints that might be given, in answer to inquiring friends. I can remember when they would have saved me some anguish of spirit; and they may be of some use to others now. I write, then, not to induce any one to talk for the sake of talking,—Heaven forbid!—but that those who are longing to say something should not fancy the obstacles insurmountable, when they are really slight.

PRINCIPLES OF GOVERNMENT.

"That liberty, or freedom, consists in having an actual share in the appointment of those who frame the laws, and who are to be the guardians of every man's life, property, and peace; for the all of one man is as dear to him as the all of another, and the poor man has an equal right, but more need, to have representatives in the legislature than the rich one. That they who have no voice nor vote in the electing of representatives do not enjoy liberty, but are absolutely enslaved to those who have votes, and to their representatives; for to be enslaved is to have governors whom other men have set over us, and be subject to laws made by the representatives of others, without having had representatives of our own to give consent in our behalf."—BENJAMIN FRANKLIN, *in Sparks's Franklin*, ii. 372.

LXXII.
WE THE PEOPLE.

I remember, that, when I went to school, I used to look with wonder on the title of a newspaper of those days which was often in the hands of one of the older scholars. I remember nothing else about the newspaper, or about the boy, except that the title of the sheet he used to unfold was "We the People;" and that he derived from it his school nickname, by a characteristic boyish parody, and was usually mentioned as "Us the Folks."

Probably all that was taught in that school, in regard to American history, was not of so much value as the permanent fixing of this phrase in our memories. It seemed very natural, in later years, to come upon my old friend "Us the Folks," reproduced in almost every charter of our national government, as thus:—

"WE THE PEOPLE of the United States, in order to form a more perfect union, establish justice, insure domestic tranquillity, provide for the common defence, promote the general welfare, and secure the blessings of liberty to ourselves and our posterity, do ordain and establish this Constitution for the United States of America."—*United States Constitution, Preamble.*

"WE THE PEOPLE of Maine do agree," etc.—*Constitution of Maine.*

"All government of right originates from THE PEOPLE, is founded in their consent, and instituted for the general good."—*Constitution of New Hampshire.*

"The body politic is formed by a voluntary association of individuals; it is a social compact, by which THE WHOLE PEOPLE covenants with each citizen, and each citizen with the whole people, that all shall be governed by certain laws for the common good."—*Constitution of Massachusetts.*

"WE THE PEOPLE of the State of Rhode Island and Providence Plantations ... do ordain and establish this constitution of government."—*Constitution of Rhode Island.*

"THE PEOPLE of Connecticut do, in order more effectually to define, secure, and perpetuate the liberties, rights, and privileges which they have derived from their ancestors, hereby ordain and establish the following constitution and form of civil government."—*Constitution of Connecticut.*

And so on through the constitutions of almost every State in the Union. Our government is, as Lincoln said, "a government of the people, by the people, and for the people." There is no escaping it. To question this is to deny the foundations of the American government. Granted that those who framed these provisions may not have understood the full extent of the principles they announced. No matter: they gave us those principles; and, having them, we must apply them.

Now, women may be voters or not, citizens or not; but that they are a part of the people, no one has denied in Christendom—however it may be in

Japan, where, as Mrs. Leonowens tells us, the census of population takes in only men, and the women and children are left to be inferred. "WE THE PEOPLE," then, includes women. Be the superstructure what it may, the foundation of the government clearly provides a place for them: it is impossible to state the national theory in such a way that it shall not include them. It is impossible to deny the natural right of women to vote, except on grounds which exclude all natural right. Dr. Bushnell, in annihilating, as he thinks, the claims of women to the ballot, annihilates the rights of the community as a whole, male or female. He may not be consistent enough to allow this, but Mr. Wasson is. That keen destructive strikes at the foundation of the building, and aims to demolish "We the people" altogether.

The fundamental charters are on our side. There are certain statute limitations which may prove greater or less. But these are temporary and trivial things, always to be interpreted, often to be modified, by reference to the principles of the Constitution. For instance, when a constitutional convention is to be held, or new conditions of suffrage to be created, the whole people should vote upon the matter, including those not hitherto enfranchised. This is the view insisted on, a few years since, by that eminent jurist, William Beach Lawrence. He maintained, in a letter to Charles Sumner and in opposition to his own party, that if the question of "negro suffrage" in the Southern States of the Union were put to vote, the colored people themselves had a natural right to vote on the question. The same is true of women. It should never be forgotten by advocates of woman suffrage, that, the deeper their reasonings go, the stronger foundation they find; and that we have always a solid fulcrum for our lever in that phrase of our charters, "We the people."

LXXIII.
THE USE OF THE DECLARATION OF INDEPENDENCE.

When young people begin to study geometry, they expect to begin with hard reasoning on the very first page. To their surprise, they find that the first few pages are not occupied by reasoning, but by a few simple, easy, and rather commonplace sentences, called "axioms," which are really a set of pegs on which all the reasoning is hung. Pupils are not expected to go back in every demonstration, and prove the axioms. If Almira Jones happens to be doing a problem at the blackboard on examination-day, at the high school, and remarks in the course of her demonstration that "things which are equal to the same thing are equal to one another," and if a sharp questioner jumps up, and says, "How do you know it?" she simply lays down her bit of chalk, and says fearlessly, "That is an axiom," and the teacher sustains her. Some things must be taken for granted.

The same service rendered by axioms in the geometry is supplied, in regard to government, by the simple principles of the Declaration of Independence. Right or wrong, they are taken for granted. Inasmuch as all the legislation of the country is supposed to be based in them,—they stating the theory of our government, while the Constitution itself only puts into organic shape the application,—we must all begin with them. It is a great convenience, and saves great trouble in all reforms. To the Abolitionists, for instance, what an inestimable labor-saving machine was the Declaration of Independence! Let them have that, and they asked no more. Even the brilliant lawyer Rufus Choate, when confronted with its plain provisions, could only sneer at them as "glittering generalities," which was equivalent to throwing down his brief, and throwing up his case. It was an admission, that, if you were so foolish as to insist on applying the first principles of the government, it was all over with him.

Now, the whole doctrine of woman suffrage follows so directly from these same political axioms, that they are especially convenient for women to have in the house. When the Declaration of Independence enumerates as among "self-evident" truths the fact of governments "deriving their just powers from the consent of the governed," then that point may be considered as settled. In this school-examination of maturer life, in this grown-up geometry-class, the student is not to be called upon by the committee to prove that. She may rightfully lay down her demonstrating chalk, and say, "That is an axiom. You admit that yourselves."

It is a great convenience. We cannot always be going back, like a Hindoo history, to the foundations of the world. Some things may be taken for granted. How this simple axiom sweeps away, for instance, the cobweb speculations as to whether voting is a natural right, or a privilege delegated by society! No matter which. Take it which way you please. That is an abstract question; but the practical question is a very simple one. "Governments owe their just powers to the consent of the governed." Either that axiom is false, or, whenever women as a class refuse their consent to the present exclusively masculine government, it can no longer claim just powers. The remedy then may be rightly demanded, which the Declaration of Independence goes on to state: "Whenever any form of government becomes destructive of these ends, it is the right of the people to alter or to abolish it, and to institute a new government, laying its foundation on such principles, and organizing its powers in such form, as to them shall seem most likely to effect their safety and happiness."

This is the use of the Declaration of Independence. Women, as a class, may not be quite ready to use it. It is the business of this book to help make them ready. But, so far as they are ready, these plain provisions are the axioms of their political faith. If the axioms mean any thing for men, they mean something for women. If men deride the axioms, it is a concession, like that of Rufus Choate, that these fundamental principles are very much in their way. But, so long as the sentences stand in that document, they can be made useful. If men try to get away from the arguments of women by saying, "But suppose we have nothing in our theory of government which requires us to grant your demand?" then women can answer, as the straightforward Traddles answered Uriah Heep, "But you have, you know: therefore, if you please, we won't suppose any such thing."

LXXIV.
THE TRADITIONS OF THE FATHERS.

It is fortunate for reformers that our fathers were clear-headed men. If they did not foresee all the applications of their own principles,—and who does?—they at least stated those principles very distinctly. This is a great convenience to us who preach, in season and out of season, on the texts they gave. Thus we are constantly told, "You are mistaken in thinking that the fathers of the Republic, when they proclaimed 'taxation without representation,' referred to individual rights. They were speaking only of national rights. They fought for national independence, not for personal rights at all."

It is in order to refute this sort of reasoning that women very often need to read American history afresh. They will soon be satisfied that such reasoning may be met with a plain, distinct denial. It is contrary to the facts. The plain truth is, that our fathers not only did not make national independence their exclusive aim, but they did not make it an aim at all until the war had actually begun. "I verily believe," wrote the brave Dr. Warren, "that the night preceding the barbarous outrages committed by the soldiery at Lexington, Concord, etc., there were not fifty people in the whole colony that ever expected any blood would be shed in the contest between us and Great Britain."

What was it, then, that had kept the colonists in a turmoil for years? Let us see.

On Monday, the 6th of March, 1775, the "freeholders and other inhabitants of Boston" met in town-meeting at Faneuil Hall, Samuel Adams being moderator. The committee appointed, the year before, to appoint an orator "to perpetuate the memory of the horrid massacre perpetrated on the evening of the 5th of March, 1770, by a party of soldiers," reported that they had selected Joseph Warren, Esq. The meeting confirmed this, and adjourned to meet at the Old South at half-past eleven, Faneuil Hall being too small. At the appointed hour, the church was crowded. The pulpit was draped in black. Forty British officers, in uniform, sat in the front pews or on the gallery-stairs. So great was the crowd, that Warren, in his orator's robe, entered the pulpit by a ladder through the window. He stood there before the representatives of royalty, and in defiance of the "Regulating Act," one of whose objects was to suppress meetings for any such purpose. What doctrines did he stand there to proclaim?

Richard Frothingham in his admirable "Life of Warren"[14] states the following as the fundamental proposition of this celebrated address:—

14. p. 430.

"That personal freedom is the right of every man, and that property, or an exclusive right to dispose of what he has honestly acquired by his own labor, necessarily arises therefrom, are truths which common-sense has placed beyond the reach of contradiction; and no man or body of men can, without being guilty of flagrant injustice, claim a right to dispose of the persons or acquisitions of any other man, or body of men, unless it can be proved that such a right had arisen from some compact between the parties in which it has been explicitly and freely granted."

"The orator then traced," says Frothingham, "the rise and progress of the aggressions on the natural right of the colonists to enjoy personal freedom and representative government." Not a word in behalf of national independence: on the contrary, he said, "An independence on Great Britain is not our aim. No: our wish is that Britain and the colonies may, like the oak and ivy, grow and increase together." What he protested against was the taking of individual property without granting the owner a voice in it, personally or through some authorized representative. And—observe!—this authorization must not be a merely negative or vaguely understood thing: it must be attested by "some compact between the parties in which it has been explicitly and freely granted." Any thing short of this was "a wicked policy," under whose influence the American had begun to behold the Briton as a ruffian, ready "first to take his property, and next, what is dearer to every virtuous man, the liberty of his country." The loss of the country's liberty was thus staked as a result, a deduction, a corollary; the original offence lay in the violation of the natural right of each to control his own personal freedom and personal property, or else, if these must be subordinated to the public good, to have at least a voice in the matter. This, and nothing else than this, was the principle of those who fought the Revolution, according to the statement of their first eminent martyr.

And it was for announcing these great doctrines, and for sealing them, three months later, with his blood, that it was said of him, on the fifth of March following, "We will erect a monument to thee in each of our grateful hearts, and to the latest ages will teach our tender infants to lisp the name of Warren with veneration and applause." That the opinions he expressed were the opinions current among the people, is proved by the general use of the cry " Liberty and Property" among all classes, at the time of the Stamp Act; a cry which puzzles the young student, until he sees that the Revolution really began with personal rights, and only slowly reached the demand for national independence. "Liberty and Property" was just as distinctly the claim of Joseph Warren as it is the claim of those women who now refuse to pay taxes because they believe in the principles of the American Revolution.

LXXV.
SOME OLD-FASHIONED PRINCIPLES.

There has been an effort, lately, to show that when our fathers said, "Taxation without representation is tyranny," they referred not to personal liberties, but to the freedom of a state from foreign power. It is fortunate that this criticism has been made, for it has led to a more careful examination of passages; and this has made it clear, beyond dispute, that the Revolutionary patriots carried their statements more into detail than is generally supposed, and affirmed their principles for individuals, not merely for the state as a whole.

In that celebrated pamphlet by James Otis, for instance, published as early as 1764, "The Rights of the Colonies Vindicated," he thus clearly lays down the rights of the individual as to taxation:—

"The very act of taxing, exercised over those who are not represented, appears to me to be depriving them of one of their most essential rights as freemen; and, if continued, seems to be, in effect, an entire disfranchisement of every civil right. For what one civil right is worth a rush, after a man's property is subject to be taken from him at pleasure, without his consent? If a man is not his own assessor, in person or by deputy, his liberty is gone, or he is entirely at the mercy of others."[15]

15. Otis: Rights of the Colonies, p. 58.

This fine statement has already done duty for liberty, in another contest; for it was quoted by Mr. Sumner in his speech of March 7, 1866, with this commentary:—

"Stronger words for universal suffrage could not be employed. His argument is, that, if men are taxed without being represented, they are deprived of essential rights; and the continuance of this deprivation despoils them of every civil right, thus making the latter depend upon the right of suffrage, which by a neologism of our day is known as a political right instead of a civil right. Then, to give point to this argument, the patriot insists that in determining taxation, 'every man must be his own assessor, in person or by deputy,' without which his liberty is entirely at the mercy of others. Here, again, in a different form, is the original thunderbolt, 'Taxation without representation is tyranny;' and the claim is made not merely for communities, but for 'every man.'"

In a similar way wrote Benjamin Franklin, some six years after, in that remarkable sheet found among his papers, and called "Declaration of those Rights of the Commonalty of Great Britain, without which they cannot be free." The leading propositions were these three:—

"That every man of the commonalty (excepting infants, insane persons, and criminals) is of common right and by the laws of God a freeman, and entitled to the free enjoyment of liberty. That liberty, or freedom, consists in having an actual share in the appointment of those who frame the laws, and who are to be the guardians of every man's life, property, and peace; for the all of one man is as dear to him as the all of another; and the poor man has an equal right, but more need, to have representatives in the legislature than the rich one. That they who have no voice nor vote in the electing of representatives do not enjoy liberty, but are absolutely enslaved to those who have votes, and to their representatives; for to be enslaved is to have governors whom other men have set over us, and be subject to laws made by the representatives of others, without having had representatives of our own to give consent in our behalf."[16]

16. Sparks's Franklin, ii. 372.

In quoting these words of Dr. Franklin, his latest biographer feels moved to add, "These principles, so familiar to us now and so obviously just, were startling and incredible novelties in 1770, abhorrent to nearly all Englishmen, and to great numbers of Americans." Their fair application is still abhorrent to a great many; or else, not willing quite to deny the theory, they limit the application by some such device as "virtual representation." Here, again, James Otis is ready for them; and Charles Sumner is ready to quote Otis, as thus:—

"No such phrase as virtual representation was ever known in law or constitution. It is altogether a subtlety and illusion, wholly unfounded and absurd. We must not be cheated by any such phantom, or any other fiction of law or politics, or any monkish trick of deceit or blasphemy."

These are the sharp words used by the patriot Otis, speaking of those who were trying to convince American citizens that they were virtually represented in Parliament. Sumner applied the same principle to the freedmen: it is now applied to women. "Taxation without representation is tyranny." "Virtual representation is altogether a subtlety and illusion, wholly unfounded and absurd." No ingenuity, no evasion, can give any escape from these plain principles. Either you must revoke the maxims of the American Revolution, or you must enfranchise woman. Stuart Mill well says in his autobiography, "The interest of woman is included in that of man exactly as much (and no more) as that of subjects in that of kings."

LXXVI.
FOUNDED ON A ROCK.

Gov. Long's letter on woman suffrage is of peculiar value, as recalling us to the simple principles of "right," on which alone the agitation can be solidly founded. The ground once taken by many, that women as women would be sure to act on a far higher political plane than men as men, is now urged less than formerly: the very mistakes and excesses of the agitation itself have partially disproved it. No cause can safely sustain itself on the hypothesis that all its advocates are saints and sages; but a cause that is based on a principle rests on a rock.

If there is any one who is recognized as a fair exponent of our national principles, it is our martyr-president Abraham Lincoln; whom Lowell calls, in his noble Commemoration Ode at Cambridge,—

"New birth of our new soil, the first American."

What President Lincoln's political principle was, we know. On his journey to Washington for his first inauguration, he said, "I have never had a feeling that did not spring from the sentiments embodied in the Declaration of Independence." To find out what was his view of those sentiments, we must go back several years earlier, and consider that remarkable letter of his to the Boston Republicans who had invited him to join them in celebrating Jefferson's birthday, in April, 1859. It was well called by Charles Sumner "a gem in political literature;" and it seems to me almost as admirable, in its way, as the Gettysburg address.

"The principles of Jefferson are the definitions and axioms of free society. And yet they are denied and evaded with no small show of success. One dashingly calls them 'glittering generalities.' Another bluntly styles them 'self-evident lies.' And others insidiously argue that they apply only to 'superior races.'"

"These expressions, differing in form, are identical in object and effect,—the subverting the principles of free government, and restoring those of classification, caste, and legitimacy. They would delight a convocation of crowned heads plotting against the people. They are the vanguard, the sappers and miners of returning despotism. We must repulse them, or they will subjugate us."

"All honor to Jefferson!—the man who, in the concrete pressure of a struggle for national independence by a single people, had the coolness, forecast, and capacity to introduce into a merely revolutionary document *an abstract truth applicable to all men and all times*, and so to embalm it there that to-day and in all coming days it shall be a rebuke and a stumbling-block to the harbingers of re-appearing tyranny and oppression."

The special "abstract truth" to which President Lincoln thus attaches a value so great, and which he pronounces "applicable to all men and all times," is evidently the assertion of the Declaration that governments derive their just powers from the consent of the governed, following the assertion that all men are born free and equal; that is, as some one has interpreted it, equally men. I do not see how any person but a dreamy recluse can deny that the strength of our republic rests on these principles; which are so thoroughly embedded in the average American mind that they take in it, to some extent, the place occupied in the average English mind by the emotion of personal loyalty to a certain reigning family. But it is impossible to defend these principles logically, as Senator Hoar has well pointed out, without recognizing that they are as applicable to women as to men. If this is the case, the claim of women rests on a right,—indeed, upon the same right which is the foundation of all our institutions.

The encouraging fact in the present condition of the whole matter is, not that we get more votes here or there for this or that form of woman suffrage—for experience has shown that there are great ups and downs in that respect; and States that at one time seemed nearest to woman suffrage, as Maine and Kansas, now seem quite apathetic. But the real encouragement is, that the logical ground is more and more conceded; and the point now usually made is, not that the Jeffersonian maxim excludes women, but that "the consent of the governed" is substantially given by the general consent of women. That this argument has a certain plausibility, may be conceded; but it is equally clear that the minority of women, those who do wish to vote, includes on the whole the natural leaders,—those who are foremost in activity of mind, in literature, in art, in good works of charity. It is, therefore, pretty sure that they only predict the opinions of the rest, who will follow them in time. And, even while waiting, it is a fair question whether the "governed" have not the right to give their votes when they wish, even if the majority of them prefer to stay away from the polls. We do not repeal our naturalization laws, although only the minority of our foreign-born inhabitants as yet take the pains to become naturalized.

LXXVII.
"THE GOOD OF THE GOVERNED."

In Paris, some years ago, I was for a time a resident in a cultivated French family, where the father was non-committal in politics, the mother and son were republicans, and the daughter was a Bonapartist. Asking the mother why the young lady thus held to a different creed from the rest, I was told that she had made up her mind that the streets of Paris were kept cleaner under the empire than since its disappearance: hence her imperialism.

I have heard American men advocate the French empire at home and abroad, without offering reasons so good as those of the lively French maiden. But I always think of her remark when the question is seriously asked, as Mr. Parkman, for instance, gravely puts it in his late rejoinder in "The North American Review,"—"The real issue is this: Is the object of government the good of the governed, or is it not?" Taken in a general sense, there is probably no disposition to discuss this conundrum, for the simple reason that nobody dissents from it. But the important point is: What does "the good of the governed" mean? Does it merely mean better street-cleaning, or something more essential?

There is nothing new in the distinction. Ever since De Tocqueville wrote his "Democracy in America," forty years ago, this precise point has been under active discussion. That acute writer himself recurs to it again and again. Every government, he points out, nominally seeks the good of the people, and rests on their will at last. But there is this difference: A monarchy organizes better, does its work better, cleans the streets better. Nevertheless De Tocqueville, a monarchist, sees this advantage in a republic, that when all this is done by the people for themselves, although the work done may be less perfect, yet the people themselves are more enlightened, better satisfied, and, in the end, their good is better served. Thus in one place he quotes a "a writer of talent" who complains of the want of administrative perfection in the United States, and says, "We are indebted to centralization, that admirable invention of a great man, for the uniform order and method which prevails alike in all the municipal budgets (of France) from the largest town to the humblest commune." But, says De Tocqueville,—

> "Whatever may be my admiration of this result, when I see the communes (municipalities) of France, with their excellent system of accounts, plunged in the grossest ignorance of their true interests, and abandoned to so incorrigible an apathy that they seem to vegetate rather than to live; when, on the other hand, I observe the activity, the information, and the spirit of enterprise which keeps society in perpetual labor, in these American townships, whose budgets are drawn up with small method and with still less uniformity,—I am struck by the spectacle; *for, to my mind, the end of a good government is to insure the welfare of a people*, and not to establish order and regularity in the midst of its misery and its distress."[17]
>
> [17]. Reeves's translation, London, 1838, vol. i. p. 97, note.

The Italics are my own; but it will be seen that he uses a phrase almost identical with Mr. Parkman's, and that he uses it to show that there is something to be looked at beyond good laws,—namely, the beneficial effect of self-government. In another place he comes back to the subject again:—

> "It is incontestable that the people frequently conducts public business very ill; but it is impossible that the lower order should take a part in public business without extending the circle of their ideas, and without quitting the ordinary routine of their mental acquirements; the humblest individual who is called upon to co-operate in the government of society acquires a certain degree of self-respect; and, as he possesses authority, he can command the services of minds much more enlightened than his own. He is canvassed by a multitude of applicants, who seek to deceive him in a thousand different ways, but who instruct him by their deceit.... Democracy does not confer the most skilful kind of government upon the people; but it produces that which the most skilful governments are frequently unable to awaken, namely, an all-pervading and restless activity, a superabundant force, and an energy which is inseparable from it, and which may, under favorable circumstances, beget the most amazing benefits. These are the true advantages of democracy."[18]
>
> [18]. Ibid., vol. ii. pp. 74, 75.

These passages and others like them are worth careful study. They clearly point out the two different standards by which we may criticise all political systems. One class of thinkers, of whom Froude is the most conspicuous, holds that the "good of the people" means good laws and good administration, and that, if these are only provided, it makes no sort of difference whether they themselves make the laws, or whether some Cæsar or Louis Napoleon provides them. All the traditions of the early and later Federalists point this way. But it has always seemed to me a theory of government essentially incompatible with American institutions. If we could once get our people saturated with it, they would soon be at the mercy of some Louis Napoleon of their own.

When President Lincoln claimed, following Theodore Parker, that ours was not merely a government for the people, but of the people and by the people as well, he recognized the other side of the matter,—that it is not only important what laws we have, but who makes the laws; and that "the end of a good government is to insure the welfare of a people," in this far wider sense. That advantage which the French writer admits in democracy, that it develops force, energy, and self-respect, is as essentially a part of "the good of the governed," as is any perfection in the details of government. And it is precisely these advantages which we expect that women, sooner or later, are to share. For them, as for men, "the good of the governed" is not genuine unless it is that kind of good which belongs to the self-governed.

LXXVIII.
RULING AT SECOND-HAND.

"Women ruled all; and ministers of state
Were at the doors of women forced to wait,—
Women, who've oft as sovereigns graced the land,
But never governed well at second-hand."

So wrote in the last century the bitter satirist Charles Churchill, and this verse will do something to keep alive his name. He touches the very kernel of the matter, and all history is on his side. The Salic Law excluded women from the throne of France,—"the kingdom of France being too noble to be governed by a woman," as it said. Accordingly the history of France shows one long line of royal mistresses ruling in secret for mischief; while more liberal England points to the reigns of Elizabeth and Anne and Victoria, to show how usefully a woman may sit upon a throne.

It was one of the merits of Margaret Fuller Ossoli, that she always pointed out this distinction. "Any woman can have influence," she said, "in some way. She need only to be a good cook or a good scold, to secure that. Woman should not merely have a share in the power of man,—for of that omnipotent Nature will not suffer her to be defrauded,—but it should be a *chartered* power, too fully recognized to be abused." We have got to meet, at any rate, this fact of feminine influence in the world. Demosthenes said that the measures which a statesman had meditated for a year might be overturned in a day by a woman. How infinitely more sensible, then, to train the woman herself in statesmanship, and give her open responsibility as well as concealed power!

The same principle of demoralizing subordination runs through the whole position of women. Many a husband makes of his wife a doll, dresses her in fine clothes, gives or withholds money according to his whims, and laughs or frowns if she asks any questions about his business. If only a petted slave, she naturally develops the vices of a slave; and when she wants more money for more fine clothes, and finds her husband out of humor, she coaxes, cheats, and lies. Many a woman half ruins her husband by her extravagance, simply because he has never told her frankly what his income is, or treated her, in money matters, like a rational being. Bankruptcy, perhaps, brings both to their senses; and thenceforward the husband discovers that his wife is a woman, not a child. But, for want of this, whole families and generations of women are trained to deception. I knew an instance where a fashionable dressmaker in New York urged an economical young girl, about to be married, to buy of her a costly *trousseau* or wedding outfit. "But I have not the money," said the maiden. "No matter," said the complaisant tempter: "I will wait four years, and send in the bill to your husband by degrees. Many ladies do it." Fancy the position of a pure young girl, wishing innocently to make herself beautiful in the eyes of her husband, and persuaded to go into his house with a trick like this upon her conscience! Yet it grows directly out of the whole theory of life which is preached to many women,—that all they seek must be won by indirect manœuvres, and not by straightforward living.

It is a mistaken system. Once recognize woman as born to be the equal, not inferior, of man, and she accepts as a right her share of the family income, of political power, and of all else that is capable of distribution. As it is, we are in danger of forgetting that woman, in mind as in body, was born to be upright. The women of Charles Reade—never by any possibility moving in a straight line where it is possible to find a crooked one—are distorted women; and Nature is no more responsible for them than for the figures produced by tight lacing and by high-heeled boots. These physical deformities acquire a charm, when the taste adjusts itself to them; and so do those pretty tricks and those interminable lies. But after all, to make a noble woman, you must give a noble training.

LXXIX.
"TOO MANY VOTERS ALREADY."

Curiously enough, the commonest argument against woman suffrage does not now take the form of an attack on women, but on men. Formerly we were told that women, as women, were incapable of voting; that they had not, as old Theophilus Parsons wrote in 1780, "a sufficient acquired discretion;" or that they had not physical strength enough; or that they were too delicate and angelic to vote. Now these remarks are waived, and the argument is: Women are certainly unfit for suffrage, since even men are unfit. It is something to have women at last recognized as politically equal to men, even if it be only in the fact of unfitness.

A spasm of re-action is just now passing over the minds of many men, especially among educated Americans, against universal suffrage. Possibly it is a re-action from that too great confidence in mere numbers which at one time prevailed. All human governments are as yet very imperfect; and, unless we view them reasonably, they are all worthless. We try them by unjust or whimsical tests. I do not see that anybody who objects to universal suffrage has any working theory to suggest as a substitute: the only plan he even implies is usually that he himself and his friends, and those whom he thinks worthy, should make the laws, or decide who should make them. From this I should utterly dissent: I should far rather be governed by the community, as a whole, than by my ablest friend and his ablest friends; for, if the whole community governs, I know it will not govern very much, and that the tendency will be towards personal freedom by common consent. But if my particular friend once begins to govern me, or I him, the love of power would be in danger of growing very much. It may be that he could be safely trusted with such authority, but I am very sure that I could not.

We shall never get much beyond that pithy question of Jefferson's, "It is said that man cannot govern himself: how, then, can he govern another?" There is absolutely no test by which we can determine, on any large scale, who are fit to exercise suffrage, and who are not. John Brown would exclude John Smith; and John Smith would wish to keep out John Brown, especially if he had inconvenient views, like him of Harper's Ferry. The safeguard of scientific legislation may be in the heads of a cultivated few, but the safeguard of personal freedom is commonly in the hands of the uncultivated many. The most moderate republican thinker might find himself under the supervision of Bismarck's police at any moment, should he visit Berlin; and how easily he might himself fall into the Bismarck way of thinking, is apparent when we consider that the excellent Dr. Joseph P. Thompson, writing from Germany, is understood gravely to recommend the exclusion of German communists from the ports of the United States. When we consider how easily the first principles of liberty might thus be sacrificed by the wise few, let us be grateful that we are protected by the presence of the multitude.

Whenever the vote goes against us, we are apt to think that there must be something wrong in the moral nature of the voters. It would be better to see if their votes cannot teach us something,—if the fact of our defeat does not show that we left out something, or failed to see some fact which our opponents saw. There could not be a plainer case of this than in recent Massachusetts elections. Many good men regarded it as a hopeless proof of ignorance or depravity in the masses, that more than a hundred thousand voters sustained General Butler for governor. For one, I regard that candidate as a demagogue, no doubt; but can anybody in Massachusetts now help seeing that the instinct which led that large mass of men to his support was in great measure a true one? Every act of the Republican legislatures since assembled has been influenced by that vague protest in behalf of State reform and economy which General Butler represented. He complicated it with other issues, very likely, and swelled the number of his supporters by unscrupulous means. It may have been very fortunate that he did not succeed; but it is fortunate that he tried, and that he found supporters. In this remarkable instance we see how the very dangers and excesses of popular suffrage work for good.

For myself, I do not see how we can have too many voters. I am very sure, that, in the long-run, voting tends to educate and enlighten men, to make them more accessible to able leadership, to give them a feeling of personal self-respect and independence. This is true not merely of Americans and Protestants, but of the foreign-born and the Roman Catholic; since experience shows that the political control and interference of the priesthood are exceedingly over-rated. I believe that the poor and the ignorant eminently need the ballot, first for self-respect, and then for self-protection; and, if so, why do not women need it for precisely the same reasons?

SUFFRAGE.

"No such phrase as virtual representation was ever known in law or constitution. It is altogether a subtlety and illusion, wholly unfounded and absurd. We must not be cheated by any such phantom or any other trick of law and politics."—JAMES OTIS, *quoted by* CHARLES SUMNER *in speech March* 7, 1866.

LXXX.
DRAWING THE LINE.

When in Dickens's "Nicholas Nickleby" the coal-heaver calls at the fashionable barber's to be shaved, the barber declines that service. The coal-heaver pleads that he saw a baker being shaved there the day before. But the barber points out to him that it is necessary to draw the line somewhere, and he draws it at bakers.

It is, doubtless, an inconvenience, in respect to woman suffrage, that so many people have their own theories as to drawing the line, and deciding who shall vote. Each has his hobby; and as the opportunity for applying it to men has passed by, each wishes to catch at the last remaining chance, and apply it to women. One believes in drawing an educational line; another, in a property qualification; another, in new restrictions on naturalization; another, in distinctions of race; and each wishes to keep women, for a time, as the only remaining victims for his experiment.

Fortunately the answer to all these objections, on behalf of woman suffrage, is very brief and simple. It is no more the business of its advocates to decide upon the best abstract basis for suffrage, than it is to decide upon the best system of education, or of labor, or of marriage. Its business is to equalize, in all these directions; nothing more. When that is done, there will be plenty still left to do, without doubt; but it will not involve the rights of women, as such. Simply to strike out the word "male" from the statute,—that is our present work. "What is sauce for the goose"—but the proverb is somewhat musty. These educational and property restrictions may be of value; but, wherever they are already removed from the men, they must be removed from women also. Enfranchise them equally, and then begin afresh, if you please, to legislate for the whole human race. What we protest against is that you should have let down the bars for one sex, and should at once become conscientiously convinced that they should be put up again for the other.

When it was, proposed to apply an educational qualification at the South after the war, the Southern white loyalists all objected to it. If you make it universal, they said, it cuts off many of the whites. If you apply it to the blacks alone, it is manifestly unjust. The case is the same with women in regard to men. As woman needs the ballot primarily to protect herself, it is manifestly unjust to restrict the suffrage for her, when man has it without restriction. If she needs protection, then she needs it all the more from being poor, or ignorant, or Irish, or black. If we do not see this, the freedwomen of the South did. There is nothing like personal wrong to teach people logic.

We hear a great deal said in dismay, and sometimes even by old abolitionists, about "increasing the number of ignorant voters." In Massachusetts, there is an educational restriction for men, such as it is; in Rhode Island, a property qualification is required for voting on certain questions. Personally, I believe with "Warrington," that, if ignorant voting be bad, ignorant nonvoting is worse; and that the enfranchised "masses," which have a legitimate outlet for their political opinions, are far less dangerous than disfranchised masses, which must rely on mobs and strikes. I will go farther, and say that I believe our Republic is, on the whole, in less danger from its poor men, who have got to stay in it and bring up their children, than from its rich men, who have always Paris and Dresden to fall back upon. As to a property qualification, there is no dispute that Rhode Island—the only New England State which has one—is the only State where votes are publicly bought and sold on any large scale. I do not see that even a poll-tax or registry-tax is of any use as a safeguard; for, if men are to be bought, the tax merely offers a more indirect and palatable form in which to pay the price. Many a man consents to have his poll-tax paid by his party or his candidate, when he would reject the direct offer of a dollar-bill.

But this is all private speculation, and has nothing to do with the woman suffrage movement. All that we can ask, as advocates of this reform, is, that the inclusion or the exclusion should be the same for both sexes. We cannot put off the equality of woman till that time, a few centuries hence, when the Social Science Association shall have succeeded in agreeing on the true basis of "scientific legislation." It is as if we urged that wives should share their husbands' dinners, and were told that the physicians had not decided whether beefsteak were wholesome. The answer is, "Beefsteak or tripe, yeast or saleratus, which you please. But, meanwhile, what is good enough for the wife is good enough for the husband."

LXXXI.
FOR SELF-PROTECTION.

I remember to have read, many years ago, the life of Sir Samuel Romilly, the English philanthropist. He was the author of more beneficent legal reforms than any man of his day, and there was in this book a long list of the changes he still meant to bring about. It struck me very much, that, among these proposed reforms, not one of any importance referred to the laws about women.

It shows—what all experience has shown—that no class or race or sex can safely trust its protection in any hands but its own. The laws of England in regard to woman were then so bad that Lord Brougham afterwards said they needed total reconstruction, if they were to be touched at all. And yet it is only since woman suffrage began to be talked about, that the work of law-reform has really taken firm hold. In many cases in America the beneficent measures are directly to be traced to some appeal from feminine advocates. Even in Canada, as stated the other day by Dr. Cameron, formerly of Toronto, the bill protecting the property of married women was passed under the immediate pressure of Lucy Stone's eloquence. And, even where this direct agency could not be traced, the general fact that the atmosphere was full of the agitation had much to do with all the reforms that took place. Legislatures, unwilling to give woman the ballot, were shamed into giving her something. The chairman of the judiciary committee in Rhode Island told me, that, until he heard women address the committee, he had not reflected upon their legal disabilities, or thought how unjust these were. While the matter was left to the other sex only, even men like Sir Samuel Romilly forgot the wrongs of woman. When she began to advocate her own cause men also waked up.

But now that they are awake, they ask, is not this sufficient? Not at all. If an agent who has cheated you surrenders reluctantly one-half your stolen goods, you do not stop there and say, "It is enough. Your intention is honorable. Please continue my agent with increased pay." On the contrary, you say, "Your admission of wrong is a plea of guilty. Give me the rest of what is mine." There is no defence like self-defence, no protection like self-protection.

All theories of chivalry and generosity and vicarious representation fall before the fact that woman has been grossly wronged by man. That being the case, the only modest and honest thing for man to do is to say, "Henceforward have a voice in making your own laws." Till this is done, she has no sure safeguard, since otherwise the same men who made the old barbarous laws may at any time restore them.

It is common to say that woman suffrage will make no great difference; for that women will think very much as men do, and it will simply double the vote without varying the result. About many matters this may be true. To be sure, it is probable that on questions of conscience, like slavery and temperance, the woman's vote would by no means coincide with man's. But grant that it would. The fact remains,—and all history shows it,—that on all that concerns her own protection a woman needs her own vote. Would a woman vote to give her husband the power of bequeathing her children to the control and guardianship of somebody else? Would a woman vote to sustain the law by which a Massachusetts chief justice bade the police take those crying children from their mother's side in the Boston court-room a few years ago, and hand them over to a comparative stranger, because that mother had married again? You might as well ask whether the colored vote would sustain the Dred Scott decision. Tariffs or banks may come or go the same, whether the voters be white or black, male or female. But, when the wrongs of an oppressed class or sex are to be righted, the ballot is the only guaranty. After they have gained a potential voice for themselves, the Sir Samuel Romillys will remember them.

LXXXII.
WOMANLY STATESMANSHIP.

The newspapers periodically express a desire to know whether women have given evidence, on the whole, of superior statesmanship to men. There are constant requests that they will define their position as to the tariff and the fisheries and the civil-service question. If they do not speak, it is naturally assumed that they will forever after hold their peace. Let us see how that matter stands.

It is said that the greatest mechanical skill in America is to be found among professional burglars who come here from England. Suppose one of these men were in prison, and we were to stand outside and taunt him through the window: "Here is a locomotive engine: why do you not mend or manage it? Here is a steam printing-press: if you know any thing, set it up for me! You a mechanic, when you have not proved that you understand any of these things? Nonsense!"

But Jack Sheppard, if he condescended to answer us at all, would coolly say, "Wait a while, till I have finished my present job. Being in prison, my first business is to get out of prison. Wait till I have picked this lock, and mined this wall; wait till I have made a saw out of a watch-spring, and a ladder out of a pair of blankets. Let me do my first task, and get out of limbo, and then see if your little printing-presses and locomotives are too puzzling for my fingers."

Politically speaking, woman is in prison, and her first act of skill must be in getting through the wall. For her there is no tariff question, no question of the fisheries. She will come to that by and by, if you please; but for the present her statesmanship must be employed nearer home. The "civil-service reform" in which she is most concerned is a reform which shall bring her in contact with the civil service. Her political creed, for the present, is limited to that of Sterne's starling in the cage,—"I can't get out." If she is supposed to have any common-sense at all, she will best show it by beginning at the point where she is, instead of at the point where somebody else is. She would indeed be as foolish as these editors think her if she now spent her brains upon the tariff question, which she cannot reach, instead of upon her own enfranchisement which she is fast reaching.

The woman suffrage movement in America, in all its stages and subdivisions, has been the work of woman. No doubt men have helped in it: much of the talking has been done by them, and they have furnished many of the printed documents. But the energy, the methods, the unwearied purpose, of the movement, have come from women: they have led in all councils; they have established the newspapers, got up the conventions, addressed the legislatures, and raised the money. Thirty years have shown, with whatever temporary variations, one vast wave of progress toward success, both in this country and in Europe. Now, success is statesmanship.

I remember well the shouts of laughter that used to greet the anti-slavery orators when they claimed that the real statesmen of the country were not the Calhouns and Websters, who spent their strength in trying to sustain slavery, and failed, but the Garrisons, who devoted their lives to its overthrow, and were succeeding. Yet who now doubts this? Tried by the same standard, the statesmanship of to-day does not lie in the men who can find no larger questions before them than those which concern the fisheries, but in the women whose far-reaching efforts will one day make every existing voting-list so much waste paper.

Of course, when the voting-lists with the women's names are ready to be printed, it will be interesting to speculate as to how these new monarchs of our destiny will use their power. For myself, a long course of observation in the anti-slavery and woman suffrage movements has satisfied me that women are not idiots, and that, on the whole, when they give their minds to a question, whether moral or practical, they understand it quite as readily as men. In the anti-slavery movement it is certain that a woman, Elizabeth Heyrick, gave the first impulse to its direct and simple solution in England; and that another woman, Mrs. Stowe, did more than any man, except perhaps Garrison and John Brown, to secure its right solution here. There was never a moment, I am confident, when any great political question growing out of the anti-slavery struggle might not have been put to vote more safely among the women of New England than among the clergy, or the lawyers, or the college-professors. If they have done so well in the last great issue, it is fair to assume, that, after they have a sufficient inducement to study out future issues, they at least will not be very much behind the men.

But we cannot keep it too clearly in view, that the whole question, whether women would vote better or worse than men on general questions, is a minor matter. It was equally a minor matter in case of the negroes. We gave the negroes the ballot, simply because they needed it for their own protection; and we shall by and by give it to women for the same reason. Tried by that test, we shall find that their statesmanship will be genuine. When they come into power, drunken husbands will no longer control their wives' earnings, and a chief justice will no longer order a child to be removed from its mother, amid its tears and outcries, merely because that mother has married again. And if, as we are constantly assured, woman's first duty is to her home and her children, she may count it a good beginning in statesmanship to secure to herself the means of protecting both. That once settled, it will be time enough to "interview" her in respect to the proper rate of duty on pig-iron.

LXXXIII.
TOO MUCH PREDICTION.

"Seek not to proticipate," says Mrs. Gamp, the venerable nurse in "Martin Chuzzlewit"—"but take 'em as they come, and as they go." I am persuaded that our woman-suffrage arguments would be improved by this sage counsel, and that at present we indulge in too many bold anticipations.

Is there not altogether too much tendency to predict what women will do when they vote? Could that good time come to-morrow, we should be startled to find to how many different opinions and "causes" the new voters were already pledged. One speaker wishes that women should be emancipated, because of the fidelity with which they are sure to support certain desirable measures, as peace, order, freedom, temperance, righteousness, and judgment to come. Then the next speaker has his or her schedule of political virtues, and is equally confident that women, if once enfranchised, will guarantee clear majorities for them all. The trouble is, that we thus mortgage this new party of the future, past relief, beyond possibility of payment, and incur the ridicule of the unsanctified by committing our cause to a great many contradictory pledges.

I know an able and high-minded woman of foreign birth, who courageously, but as I think mistakenly, calls herself an atheist, and who has for years advocated woman-suffrage as the only antidote to the rule of the clergy. On the other hand, an able speaker in the late Boston convention advocated the same thing as the best way of defeating atheism, and securing the positive assertion of religion by the community. Both cannot be correct: neither is entitled to speak for woman. That being the case, would it not be better to keep clear of this dangerous ground of prediction, and keep to the argument based on rights and needs? If our theory of government be worth any thing, woman has the same right to the ballot that man has: she certainly needs it as much for self-defence. How she will use it, when she gets it, is her own affair. It may be that she will use it more wisely than her brothers; but I am satisfied to believe that she will use it as well. Let us not attribute infallible wisdom and virtue, even to women; for, as dear Mrs. Poyser says in Adam Bede, "God Almighty made some of 'em foolish, to match the men."

It is common to assume, for instance, that all women by nature favor peace; and that, even if they do not always seem to promote it in their social walk and conversation, they certainly will in their political. When we consider how all the pleasing excitements, achievements, and glories of war, such as they are, accrue to men only, and how large a part of the miseries are brought home to women, it might seem that their vote on this matter, at least, would be a sure thing. Thus far the theory: the fact being that we have but just emerged from a civil war which convulsed the nation, and cost half a million lives; and which was, from the very beginning, fomented, stimulated, and applauded, at least on one side, by the united voice of the women. It will be generally admitted by those who know, that, but for the women of the seceding States, the war of the Rebellion would have been waged more feebly, been sooner ended, and far more easily forgotten. Nay, I was told a few days since by an able Southern lawyer, who was long the mayor of one of the largest Southern cities, that in his opinion the practice of duelling—which is an epitome of war—owes its continued existence at the South to a sustaining public sentiment among the women.

Again, where the sympathy of women is wholly on the side of right, it is by no means safe to assume that their mode of enforcing that sentiment will be equally judicious. Take, for instance, the temperance cause. It is usual to assume that women are a unit on that question. When we look at the two extremes of society,—the fine lady pressing wine upon her New Year's visitors, and the Irishwoman laying in a family supply of whiskey to last over Sunday,—the assumption seems hasty. But grant it. Is it equally sure, that when woman takes hold of that most difficult of all legislation, the license and prohibitory laws, she will handle them more wisely than men have done? Will her more ardent zeal solve the problem on which so much zeal has already been lavished in vain? In large cities, for instance, where there is already more law than can be enforced, will her additional ballots afford the means to enforce it? It may be so; but it seems wiser not to predict nor to anticipate, but to wait and hope.

It is no reproach on woman to say that she is not infallible on particular questions. There is much reason to suppose that in politics, as in every other sphere, the joint action of the sexes will be better and wiser than that of either singly. It seems obvious that the experiment of republican government will be more fairly tried when one-half the race is no longer disfranchised. It is quite certain, at any rate, that no class can trust its rights to the mercy and chivalry of any other, but that, the weaker it is, the more it needs all political aids and securities for self-protection. Thus far, we are on safe ground; and here, as it seems to me, the claim for suffrage may securely rest. To go farther in our assertions, seems to me unsafe, although many of our wisest and most eloquent may differ from me; and, the nearer we approach success, the more important it is to look to our weapons. It is a plausible and tempting argument, to claim suffrage for woman on the ground that she is an angel; but I think it will prove wiser, in the end, to claim it for her as being human.

LXXXIV.
FIRST-CLASS CARRIAGES.

In a hotly contested municipal election, the other day, an active political manager was telling me his tactics. "We have to send carriages for some of the voters," he said. "First-class carriages! If we undertake to wait on 'em, we must do it in good shape, and not leave the best carriages to be hired by the other party."

I am not much given to predicting just what will happen when women vote; but I confidently assert that they will be taken to the polls, if they wish, in first-class carriages. If the best horses are to be harnessed, and the best cushions selected, and every panel of the coach rubbed till you can see your face in it, merely to accommodate some elderly man who lives two blocks away, and could walk to the polls very easily, then how much more will these luxuries be placed at the service of every woman, young or old, whose presence at the polls is made doubtful by mud, or snow, or the prospect of a shower!

But the carriage is only the beginning of the polite attentions that will soon appear. When we see the transformation undergone by every ferry-boat and every railway-station, so soon as it comes to be frequented by women, who can doubt that voting-places will experience the same change? They will soon have—at least in the "ladies' department,"—elegance instead of discomfort, beauty for ashes, plenty of rocking-chairs, and no need of spittoons.[19] Very possibly they may have all the modern conveniences and inconveniences,—furnace-registers, tea-kettles, Washington-pies, and a young lady to give checks for bundles. Who knows what elaborate comforts, what queenly luxuries, may be offered to women at voting-places, when the time has finally arrived to sue for their votes?

19. Since this was written, the legislature of Massachusetts has passed, with little opposition, a law prohibiting smoking at voting-places,—an explicit fulfilment of this prophecy.

The common impression has always been quite different from this. People look at the coarseness and dirt now visible at so many voting-places, and say, "Would you expose women to all that?" But these places are not dirtier than a railway smoking-car; and there is no more coarseness than in any ferry-boat which is, for whatever reason, used by men only. You do not look into those places, and say with indignation, "Never, if I can help it, shall my wife or my beloved great-grandmother travel by steamboat or by rail!" You know that with these exemplary relatives will enter order and quiet, carpets and curtains, brooms and dusters. Why should it be otherwise with wardrooms and town-halls?

There is not an atom more of intrinsic difficulty in providing a decorous ladies' room for a voting-place, than for a post-office or a railway-station; and it is as simple a thing to vote a ticket as to buy one. This being thus easily practicable, all men will desire to provide it. And the example of the first-class carriages shows that the parties will vie with each other in these pleasing arrangements. They will be driven to it, whether they wish it or not. The party which has most consistently and resolutely kept woman away from the ballot-box will be the very party compelled, for the sake of self-preservation, to make her "rights" agreeable to her when once she gets them. A few stupid or noisy men may indeed try to make the polls unattractive to her, the very first time; but the result of this little experiment will be so disastrous that the offenders will be sternly suppressed by their own party-leaders, before another election-day comes. It will soon become clear, that, of all possible ways of losing votes, the surest lies in treating women rudely.

Lucy Stone tells a story of a good man in Kansas, who, having done all he could to prevent women from being allowed to vote on school questions, was finally comforted, when that measure passed, by the thought that he should at least secure his wife's vote for a pet schoolhouse of his own. Election-day came, and the newly enfranchised matron showed the most culpable indifference to her privileges. She made breakfast as usual, went about her housework, and did on that perilous day precisely the things that her anxious husband had always predicted that women never would do under such circumstances. His hints and advice found no response; and nothing short of the best pair of horses and the best wagon finally sufficed to take the farmer's wife to the polls. I am not the least afraid that women will find voting a rude or disagreeable arrangement. There is more danger of their being treated too well, and being too much attacked and allured by these cheap cajoleries. But women are pretty shrewd, and can probably be trusted to go to the polls, even in first-class carriages.

LXXXV.
EDUCATION *via* SUFFRAGE.

I know a rich bachelor of large property, who fatigues his friends by perpetual denunciations of every thing American, and especially of universal suffrage. He rarely votes; and I was much amazed, when the popular vote was to be taken on building an expensive schoolhouse, to see him go to the polls, and vote in the affirmative. On being asked his reason, he explained, that, while we labored under the calamity of universal (male) suffrage, he thought it best to mitigate its evils by educating the voters. In short, he wished, as Mr. Lowe said in England when the last Reform Bill passed, "to prevail upon our future masters to learn their alphabets."

These motives may not be generous; but the schoolhouses, when they are built, are just as useful. Even girls get the benefit of them, though the long delay in many places before girls got their share came in part from the want of this obvious stimulus. It is universal male suffrage that guarantees schoolhouse and school. The most selfish man understands that argument: "We must educate the masses, if it is only to keep them from our throats."

But there is a wider way in which suffrage guarantees education. At every election-time, political information is poured upon the whole voting community, till it is deluged. Presses run night and day to print newspaper extras; clerks sit up all night to frank congressional speeches; the most eloquent men in the community expound the most difficult matters to the ignorant. Of course each party affords only its own point of view; but every man has a neighbor who is put under treatment by some other party, and who is constantly attacking all who will listen to his provoking and pestilent counter-statements. All the common-school education of the United States does not equal the education of election-day; and, as in some States elections are held very often, this popular university seems to be kept in session almost the whole year round. The consequence is a remarkable average popular knowledge of political affairs,—a training which American women now miss, but which will come to them with the ballot.

And in still another way, there will be an education coming to woman from the right of suffrage. It will come from her own sex, proceeding from highest to lowest. We often hear it said, that, after enfranchisement, the more educated women will not vote, while the ignorant will. But Mrs. Howe admirably pointed out, at a Philadelphia convention, that, the moment women have the ballot, it will become the pressing duty of the more educated women, even in self-protection, to train the rest. The very fact of the danger will be a stimulus to duty, with women, as it already is with men.

It has always seemed to me rather childish, in a man of superior education, or talent, or wealth, to complain that when election-day comes he has no more votes than the man who plants his potatoes or puts in his coal. The truth is, that under the most thorough system of universal suffrage the man of wealth or talent or natural leadership has still a disproportionate influence, still casts a hundred votes where the poor or ignorant or feeble man throws but one. Even the outrages of New York elections turned out to be caused by the fact that the leading rogues had used their brains and energy, while the men of character had not. When it came to the point, it was found that a few caricatures by Nast and a few columns of figures in the Times were more than a match for all the repeaters of the ring. It is always so. Andrew Johnson, with all the patronage of the nation, had not the influence of "Nasby" with his one newspaper. The whole Chinese question was perceptibly and instantly modified when Harte wrote "The Heathen Chinee."

These things being so, it indicates feebleness or dyspepsia when an educated man is heard whining, about election-time, with his fears of ignorant voting. It is his business to enlighten and control that ignorance. With a voice and a pen at his command, with a town-hall in every town for the one, and a newspaper in every village for the other, he has such advantages over his ignorant neighbors that the only doubt is whether his privileges are not greater than he deserves. For one, in writing for the press, I am impressed by the undue greatness, not by the littleness, of the power I wield. And what is true of men will be true of women. If the educated women of America have not brains or energy enough to control, in the long-run, the votes of the ignorant women around them, they will deserve a severe lesson, and will be sure, like the men in New York, to receive it. And thenceforward they will educate and guide that ignorance, instead of evading or cringing before it.

But I have no fear about the matter. It is a libel on American women to say that they will not go anywhere or do any thing which is for the good of their children and their husbands. Travel West on any of our great lines of railroad, and see what women undergo in transporting their households to their new homes. See the watching and the feeding, and the endless answers to the endless questions, and the toil to keep little Sarah warm, and little Johnny cool, and the baby comfortable. What a hungry, tired, jaded, forlorn mass of humanity it is, as the sun rises on it each morning, in the soiled and breathless railway-car! Yet that household group is America in the making; those are the future kings and queens, the little princes and princesses, of this land. Now, is the mother who has undergone for the transportation of these children all this enormous labor, to shrink at her journey's end from the slight additional labor of going to the polls to vote whether those little ones shall have schools or rumshops? The thought is an absurdity. A few fine ladies in cities will fear to spoil their silk dresses, as a few foppish gentlemen now fear for their broadcloth. But the mass of intelligent American women will vote, as do the mass of men.

LXXXVI.
"OFF WITH HER HEAD!"

In "Alice's Adventures in Wonderland," the Queen of Hearts settles all disputes at croquet by ordering somebody's head to be taken off. It is the old royal remedy. The Roman Tarquin, when his son sent to ask him the best way of reducing a discontented city, merely slashed off the heads of the tallest poppies, as he walked in the garden. The young man took the hint, and performed a similar process upon the leading citizens.

Every year makes it plainer that the community must imitate Tarquinius Superbus and the Queen of Hearts if it wishes to get rid of the woman suffrage movement. So long as every woman favors it whenever she gets her head above a certain point, so long those conspicuous heads must be recognized. You must either put them on the voting-list, or on the list ordered for immediate execution: there is no middle ground.

There are the women who write books, for instance. When authorship first came up among the women of America, they not only claimed nothing more than the mere privilege of having brains, but they almost apologized for that. Their early authors, as Mrs. Child and Mrs. Leslie, had a way of preparing a cookery-book apiece, as a propitiation to the tyrant man, before proceeding to what is called "the intellectual feast." They held, with Miss Bremer, that you can get any thing you like from a man if you will only have something nice to pop into his mouth. Mrs. Sarah J. Hale, in her "Woman's Record," published twenty years ago, adopted a different form of submission. She seemed very anxious to prove that women had taken a prominent part in the world; but also to show, that, if they were only forgiven for this, they would never, never, never make themselves any more prominent. It is but within a few years that literary women have dared to go beyond literature, and ask for a vote besides.

But now, with what a terrible confidence they come to the demand for suffrage when they acquire voice enough to make themselves heard! Mrs. Stowe helps to free Uncle Tom in his cabin, and then strikes for the freedom of women in her own "Hearth and Home." Mrs. Howe writes the "Battle Hymn of the Republic," and keeps on writing more battle-hymns in behalf of her own sex. Miss Alcott not only delineates "Little Women," but wishes to emancipate them. Miss Phelps desires to see the "Gates Ajar" for her sex, both in heaven and on earth. Mrs. Child, who risked her literary popularity in early life by her "Appeal for that Class of Americans called Africans," was as ready to risk it again for that class of Americans called women.

Of course, there are social circles in America where all desire for leadership on the part of literary women would be repudiated; nay, where the fact that a woman had written a book would imply a loss of caste. When Karl von Beethoven signed himself "*Gutsbesitzer*," or "land proprietor," his brother Ludwig signed himself "*Hirnbesitzer*," or "proprietor of a brain." Posterity remembers only the great musical composer; yet, doubtless, to the society of that period, the stupid elder brother was by far the greater man. Such perversities cannot be helped; but I write for reasonable people. Among the women who dance the German, woman suffrage may be just now unpopular; but the women who translate German will in the long-run have most influence, and their verdict seems to tend the other way. It is said that the leading dancer among the young men of one of our cities was transformed into an equally prominent lawyer by a single suggestion from an elder sister, that it was "better to be a man of books than a man of toes." It is likely that America will be more influenced at last by the women of heads than by the women of heels.

LXXXVII.
FOLLOW YOUR LEADERS.

"There go thirty thousand men," shouted the Portuguese, as Wellington, with a few staff-officers, rode along the mountain-side. The action of the leaders' minds, in any direction, has a value out of all proportion to their numbers. In a campaign, there is a council of officers,—Grant and Sherman and Sheridan perhaps. They are but a trifling minority, yet what they plan the whole army will do; and such is the faith in a real leader, that, were all the restraints of discipline for the moment relaxed, the rank and file would still follow his judgment. What a few general officers see to be the best to-day, the sergeants and corporals and private soldiers will usually see to be best to-morrow.

In peace, also, there is a silent leadership; only that in peace, as there is more time to spare, the leaders are expected to persuade the rank and file, instead of commanding them. Yet it comes to the same thing in the end. The movement begins with certain guides, and, if you wish to know the future, keep your eye on them. If you wish to know what is already decided, ask the majority; but, if you wish to find out what is likely to be done next, ask the leaders.

It is constantly said that the majority of women do not yet desire to vote, and it is true. But, to find out whether they are likely to wish for it, we must keep our eyes on the women who lead their sex. The representative women, —those who naturally stand for the rest, those most eminent for knowledge and self-devotion,—how do they view the thing? The rank and file do not yet demand the ballot, you say; but how is it with the general officers?

Now, it is a remarkable fact, about which those who have watched this movement for twenty years can hardly be mistaken, that almost any woman who reaches a certain point of intellectual or moral development will presently be found desiring the ballot for her sex. If this be so, it predicts the future. It is the judgment of Grant and Sherman and Sheridan as against that of the average private soldier of the Two Hundredth Infantry. Set aside, if you please, the specialists of this particular agitation,—those who were first known to the public through its advocacy. There is no just reason why they should be set aside, yet concede that for a moment. The fact remains that the ablest women in the land—those who were recognized as ablest in other spheres, before they took this particular duty upon them—are extremely apt to assume this cross when they reach a certain stage of development.

When Margaret Fuller first came forward into literature, she supposed that literature was all she wanted. It was not till she came to write upon woman's position that she discovered what woman needed. Clara Barton, driving her ambulance or her supply-wagon at the battle's edge, did not foresee, perhaps, that she should make that touching appeal, when the battle was over, imploring her own enfranchisement from the soldiers she had befriended. Lydia Maria Child, Julia Ward Howe, Harriet Beecher Stowe, Louisa Alcott, came to the claim for the ballot earlier than a million others, because they were the intellectual leaders of American womanhood. They saw farthest, because they were in the highest place. They were the recognized representatives of their sex before they gave in their adhesion to the new demand. Their judgment is as the judgment of the council of officers; while Flora McFlimsey's opinion is as the opinion of John Smith, unassigned recruit. But, if the generals make arrangements for a battle, the chance is that John Smith will have to take a hand in it, or else run away.

It is a rare thing for the petition for suffrage from any town to comprise the majority of women in that town. It makes no difference: if there are few women in the town who want to vote, there is as much propriety in their voting as if there were ten millions, so long as the majority are equally protected in their right to stay at home. But, when the names of petitioners come to be weighed as well as counted, the character, the purity, the intelligence, the social and domestic value, of the petitioners, is seldom denied. The women who wish to vote are not the idle, the ignorant, the narrow-minded, or the vicious; they are not "the dangerous classes:" they represent the best class in the community, when tried by the highest standard. They are the natural leaders. What they now see to be right, will also be perceived even by the foolish and the ignorant by and by.

In a poultry-yard in spring, when the first brood of ducklings go toddling to the water-side, no doubt all the younger or feebler broods, just hatched out of similar eggs, think these innovators dreadfully mistaken. "You are out of place," they feebly pipe. "See how happy we are in our safe nests. Perhaps, by and by, when properly introduced into society, we may run about a little on land, but to swim!—never!" Meanwhile their elder kindred are splashing and diving in ecstasy; and, so surely as they are born ducklings, all the rest will swim in their turn. The instinct of the first duck solves the problem for all the rest. It is a mere question of time. Sooner or later, all the broods in the most conservative yard will follow their leaders.

LXXXVIII.
HOW TO MAKE WOMEN UNDERSTAND POLITICS.

An English member of Parliament said in a speech, some years ago, that the stupidest man had a clearer understanding of political questions than the brightest woman. He did not find it convenient to say what must be the condition of a nation which for many years has had a woman for its sovereign; but he certainly said bluntly what many men feel. It is not indeed very hard to find the source of this feeling. It is not merely that women are inexperienced in questions of finance or administrative practice, for many men are equally ignorant of these. But it is undoubtedly true of a large class of more fundamental questions,—as, for instance, of some now pending at Washington,—which even many clear-headed women find it hard to understand, while men of far less general training comprehend them entirely. Questions of the distribution of power, for instance, between the executive, judicial, and legislative branches of government,—or between the United States government and those of the separate States,—belong to the class I mean. Many women of great intelligence show a hazy indistinctness of views when the question arises whether it is the business of the General Government to preserve order at the voting-places at a congressional election, for instance, as the Republicans hold; or whether it should be left absolutely in the hands of the State officials, as the Democrats maintain. Most women would probably say that so long as order was preserved, it made very little difference who did it. Yet, if one goes into a shoe-shop or a blacksmith's shop, one may hear just these questions discussed in all their bearings by uneducated men, and it will be seen that they involve a principle. Why is this difference? Does it show some constitutional inferiority in women, as to this particular faculty?

The question is best solved by considering a case somewhat parallel. The South Carolina negroes were considered very stupid, even by many who knew them; and they certainly were densely ignorant on many subjects. Put face to face with a difficult point of finance legislation, I think they would have been found to know even less about it than I do. Yet the abolition of slavery was held in those days by many great statesmen to be a subject so difficult that they shrank from discussing it; and nevertheless I used to find that these ignorant men understood it quite clearly in all its bearings. Offer a bit of sophistry to them, try to blind them with false logic on this subject, and they would detect it as promptly, and answer it as keenly, as Garrison or Phillips would have done; and, indeed, they would give very much the same answers. What was the reason? Not that they were half wise and half stupid; but that they were dull where their own interests had not trained them, and they were sharp and keen where their own interests were concerned.

I have no doubt that it will be so with women when they vote. About some things they will be slow to learn; but, about all that immediately concerns themselves, they will know more at the very beginning than many wise men have learned since the world began. How long it took for English-speaking men to correct, even partially, the iniquities of the old common law!—but a parliament of women would have set aside at a single sitting the alleged right of the husband to correct his wife with a stick no bigger than his thumb. It took the men of a certain State of this Union a good many years to see that it was an outrage to confiscate to the State one-half the property of a man who died childless, leaving his widow only the other half; but a legislature of women would have annihilated that enormity by a single day's work. I have never seen reason to believe that women on general questions would act more wisely or more conscientiously, as a rule, than men: but self-preservation is a wonderful quickener of the brain; and, in all questions bearing on their own rights and opportunities as women, it is they who will prove shrewd and keen, and men who will prove obtuse, as indeed they have usually been.

Another point that adds force to this is the fact that wherever women, by their special position, have more at stake than usual in public affairs, even as now organized, they are apt to be equal to the occasion. When the men of South Carolina were ready to go to war for the "States-Rights" doctrines of Calhoun, the women of that State had also those doctrines at their fingers'-ends. At Washington, where politics make the breath of life, you will often find the wives of members of Congress following the debates, and noting every point gained or lost, because these are matters in which they and their families are personally concerned; and, as for that army of women employed in the "departments" of the government, they are politicians every one, because their bread depends upon it.

The inference is, that, if women as a class are now unfitted for politics, it is because they have not that pressure of personal interest and responsibility by which men are unconsciously trained. Give this, and self-interest will do the rest; aided by that power of conscience and affection which is certainly not less in them than in men, even if we claim no more. A young lady of my acquaintance opposed woman suffrage in conversation on various grounds, one of which was that it would, if enacted, compel her to read the newspapers, which she greatly disliked. I pleaded that this was not a fatal objection; since many men voted "early and often" without reading them, and in fact without knowing how to read at all. She said, in reply, that this might do for men, but that women were far more conscientious, and, if they were once compelled to vote, they would wish to know what they were voting for. This seemed to me to contain the whole philosophy of the matter; and I respected the keenness of her suggestion, though it led me to an opposite conclusion.

LXXXIX.
"INFERIOR TO MAN, AND NEAR TO ANGELS."

If it were anywhere the custom to disfranchise persons of superior virtue because of their virtue, and to present others with the ballot, simply because they had been in the State Prison,—then the exclusion of women from political rights would be a high compliment, no doubt. But I can find no record in history of any such legislation, unless so far as it is contained in the doubtful tradition of the Tuscan city of Pistoia, where men are said to have been ennobled as a punishment for crime. Among us crime may often be a covert means of political prominence, but it is not the ostensible ground; nor are people habitually struck from the voting-lists for performing some rare and eminent service, such as saving human life, or reading every word of a Presidential message. If a man has been President of the United States, we do not disfranchise him thenceforward; if he has been governor, we do not declare him thenceforth ineligible to the office of United States senator. On the contrary, the supposed reward of high merit is to give higher civic privileges. Sometimes these are even forced on unwilling recipients, as when Plymouth Colony in 1633 imposed a fine of twenty pounds on any one who should refuse the office of governor.

It is utterly contrary to all tradition and precedent, therefore, to suppose that women have been hitherto disfranchised because of any supposed superiority. Indeed, the theory is self-annihilating, and involves all supporters in hopeless inconsistency. Thus the Southern slaveholders were wont to argue that a negro was only blest when a slave, and there was no such inhumanity as to free him. Then, if a slave happened to save his master's life, he was rewarded by emancipation immediately, amid general applause. The act refuted the theory. And so, every time we have disfranchised a rebel, or presented some eminent foreigner with the freedom of a city, we have recognized that enfranchisement, after all, means honor, and disfranchisement implies disgrace.

I do not see how any woman can help a thrill of indignation, when she first opens her eyes to the fact that it is really contempt, not reverence, that has so long kept her sex from an equal share of legal, political, and educational rights. In spite of the duty paid to individual women as mothers, in spite of the reverence paid by the Greeks and the Germanic races to certain women as priestesses and sibyls, the fact remains that this sex has been generally recognized, in past ages of the human race, as stamped by hopeless inferiority, not by angelic superiority. This is carried so far, that a certain taint of actual inferiority is held to attach to women, in barbarous nations. Among certain Indian tribes, the service of the gods is defiled if a woman but touches the implements of sacrifice; and a Turk apologizes to a Christian physician for the mention of the women of his family, in the phrases used to soften the mention of any degrading creature. Mr. Leland tells us, that, among the English gypsies, any object that a woman treads upon, or sweeps with the skirts of her dress, is destroyed or made away with in some way, as unfit for use. In reading the history of manners, it is easy to trace the steps from this degradation up to the point now attained, such as it is. Yet even the habit of physiological contempt is not gone, as readers of late controversies on "Sex in Education" know full well; and I do not see how any one can read history without seeing, all around us, in society, education, and politics, the tradition of inferiority. Many laws and usages which in themselves might not strike all women as intrinsically worth striving for—as the exclusion of women from colleges or from the ballot-box—assume great importance to a woman's self-respect, when she sees in these the plain survival of the same contempt that once took much grosser forms.

And it must be remembered that in civilized communities the cynics, who still frankly express this utter contempt, are better friends to women than the flatterers, who conceal it in the drawing-room, and only utter it freely in the lecture-room, the club, and the North American Review. Contempt at least arouses pride and energy. To be sure, in the face of history, the contemptuous tone in regard to women seems to me untrue, unfair, and dastardly; but, like any other extreme injustice, it leads to re-action. It helps to awaken women from that shallow dream of self-complacency into which flattery lulls them. There is something tonic in the manly arrogance of Fitzjames Stephen, who derides the thought that the marriage-contract can be treated as in any sense a contract between equals; but there is something that debilitates in the dulcet counsel given by an anonymous gentleman, in an old volume of the Ladies' Magazine that lies before me, "She ought to present herself as a being made to please, to love, and to seek support; *a being inferior to man, and near to angels.*"

www.ingramcontent.com/pod-product-compliance
Lightning Source LLC
Chambersburg PA
CBHW081616100526
44590CB00021B/3460